Stahl's Illustrated
Substance Use and Impulsive Disorders

Stephen M. Stahl
University of California at San Diego

Meghan M. Grady
Neruoscience Education Institute

Nancy Muntner
Illustrations

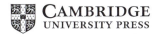

CAMBRIDGE UNIVERSITY PRESS
Cambridge, New York, Melbourne, Madrid, Cape Town, Singapore,
São Paulo, Delhi, Dubai

Cambridge University Press
The Edinburgh Building, Cambridge CB2 8RU, UK

Published in the United States of America by
Cambridge University Press, New York

www.cambridge.org
Information on this title: www.cambridge.org/9781107674530

© Neuroscience Education Institute 2012

This publication is in copyright. Subject to statutory exception
and to the provisions of relevant collective licensing agreements,
no reproduction of any part may take place without the written
permission of Cambridge University Press.

First published 2012

Printed and Bound in the United Kingdom by the MPG Books Group

A catalog record for this publication is available from the British Library.

Library of Congress Cataloging in Publication data

ISBN 978-1-107-67453-0 Paperback

Cambridge University Press has no responsibility for the
persistence or accuracy of URLs for external or third-party Internet
Web sites referred to in this publication and does not guarantee that
any content on such Web sites is, or will remain, accurate or
appropriate.

Every effort has been made in preparing this book to provide accurate and
up-to-date information that is in accord with accepted standards and
practice at the time of publication. Although case histories are drawn
from actual cases, every effort has been made to disguise the identities of
the individuals involved. Nevertheless, the authors, editors, and publishers
can make no warranties that the information contained herein is totally
free from error, not least because clinical standards are constantly
changing through research and regulation. The authors, editors, and
publishers therefore disclaim all liability for direct or consequential
damages resulting from the use of material contained in this book. Readers
are strongly advised to pay careful attention to information provided by
the manufacturer of any drugs or equipment that they plan to use.

PREFACE

These books are designed to be fun, with all concepts illustrated by full-color images and the text serving as a supplement to figures, images, and tables. The visual learner will find that this book makes psychopharmacological concepts easy to master, while the non-visual learner may enjoy a shortened text version of complex psychopharmacological concepts. Each chapter builds upon previous chapters, synthesizing information from basic biology and diagnostics to building treatment plans and dealing with complications and comorbidities.

Novices may want to approach this book by first looking through all the graphics, gaining a feel for the visual vocabulary on which our psychopharmacological concepts rely. After this once-over glance, we suggest going back through the book to incorporate the images with supporting text. Learning from visual concepts and textual supplements should reinforce one another, providing you with solid conceptual understanding at each step along the way.

Readers more familiar with these topics should find that going back and forth between images and text provides an interaction with which to vividly conceptualize complex psychopharmacology. You may find yourself using this book frequently to refresh your psychopharmacological knowledge. And you will hopefully refer your colleagues to this desk reference.

This book is intended as a conceptual overview of different topics; we provide you with a visual-based language to incorporate the rules of psychopharmacology at the expense of discussing the exceptions to these rules. The References section at the end gives you a good start for more in-depth learning about particular concepts presented here.

When you come across an abbreviation you don't understand, you can refer to the Abbreviations list in the back. *Stahl's Essential Psychopharmacology, 3rd Edition*, and *Stahl's Essential Psychopharmacology: The Prescriber's Guide, 4th Edition*, can be helpful supplementary tools for more in-depth information on particular topics in this book. Now you can also search topics in psychopharmacology on the Neuroscience Education Institute's Web site (www.neiglobal.com) for lectures, courses, slides, and related articles.

Whether you are a novice or an experienced psychopharmacologist, this book will hopefully lead you to think critically about the complexities involved in psychiatric disorders and their treatments.

Best wishes for your educational journey into the fascinating field of psychopharmacology!

Stephen M. Stahl

Table of Contents

Preface	iii
CME Information	vii
Objectives	xi
Chapter 1: Substance Use and Addiction: An Overview	1
Chapter 2: The Neurobiology of Reward and Drug Addiction	11
Chapter 3: Alcohol	35
Chapter 4: Opioids	61
Chapter 5: Nicotine	77
Chapter 6: Stimulants	99
Chapter 7: Marijuana	113
Chapter 8: Other Drugs of Abuse	121
Chapter 9: Psychosocial Treatment for Substance Use Disorders	133
Chapter 10: Disorders of Impulsivity and Compulsivity	143
Summary	157
Abbreviations	158
References	159
Index	165
CME: Posttest and Certificate	171

CME Information

Overview
In this book, we provide the biological background that will enable the reader to understand not only how chronic drug exposure is thought to alter reward circuitry, but also how currently available treatments for various substance use disorders work in the brain. We also review screening, treatment, and general management strategies for patients with addiction to various substances of abuse. In addition, we briefly touch on impulse control disorders that may have neurobiological similarities to drug addiction.

Target Audience
This activity has been developed for psychiatrists specializing in psychopharmacology. There are no prerequisites. All other health care providers who are interested in psychopharmacology are welcome for advanced study, especially primary care physicians, nurse practitioners, psychologists, and pharmacists.

Statement of Need
The following unmet needs and professional practice gaps regarding substance use were revealed following a critical analysis of activity feedback, expert faculty assessment, literature review, and through new medical knowledge:

- Substance use disorders (SUDs) are associated with significant medical, psychiatric, social, and economic consequences for both the individual and society
- Individuals who abuse and/or are dependent on substances generally need treatment to remit, making active participation of the clinician integral to the patient's successful recovery
- In a 2011 NEI Survey, 40% of respondents indicated a lack of competence in terms of treating alcohol dependence, 26% indicated lack of competence conducting a brief intervention for patients with SUDs, and 35% indicated lack of competence treating patients with SUDs and psychiatric illness

To help address clinician performance gaps with respect to diagnosis and treatment of substance use disorders, quality improvement efforts need to provide education regarding (1) screening methods for substance use disorders and how to implement them for all patients; (2) appropriate advice and management strategies for patients at risk of substance use disorders; (3) current and emerging treatment strategies for various substance use disorders; (4) techniques for monitoring patient progress and addressing adherence concerns; and (5) underlying risk factors for substance use disorders, including clinical, behavioral, and neurobiological factors.

Learning Objectives
After completing this activity, participants should be better able to:

- Apply evidence-based screening methods to identify patients who are dependent or at risk of becoming dependent on substances of abuse
- Provide preventive counseling and brief interventions for patients at risk of becoming addicted/dependent
- Apply evidence-based treatment strategies to individuals with substance use disorders
- Include strategies for monitoring improvement and addressing adherence as part of the treatment plan for patients with substance use disorders
- Recognize the clinical, behavioral, and neurobiological links between substance use disorders and other disorders of impulsivity

Accreditation and Credit Designation Statements
The Neuroscience Education Institute is accredited by the Accreditation Council for Continuing Medical Education to provide continuing medical education for physicians.

The Neuroscience Education Institute designates this enduring material for a maximum of 6.0 AMA PRA Category 1 Credits™. Physicians should claim only the credit commensurate with the extent of their participation in the activity.

Nurses: for all of your CNE requirements for recertification, the ANCC will accept AMA PRA Category 1 Credits™ from organizations accredited by the ACCME.

Physician Assistants: the NCCPA accepts AMA PRA Category 1 Credits™ from organizations accredited by the AMA (providers accredited by the ACCME).

A certificate of participation for completing this activity will also be available.

Activity Instructions
This CME activity is in the form of a printed monograph and incorporates instructional design to enhance your retention of the information and pharmacological concepts that are being presented. You are advised to go through the figures in this activity from beginning to end, followed by the text, and then complete the posttest and activity evaluation. The estimated time for completion of this activity is 6.0 hours.

Instructions for CME Credit
To receive your certificate of CME credit or participation, please complete the posttest and evaluation, available only online at **www.neiglobal.com/CME** (under "Book"). If a passing score of 70% or more is attained (required to receive credit), you can immediately print your certificate. There is a fee for the posttest (waived for NEI members).). If you have questions, please call 888-535-5600, or email customerservice@neiglobal.com.

NEI Disclosure Policy

It is the policy of the Neuroscience Education Institute to ensure balance, independence, objectivity, and scientific rigor in all its educational activities. Therefore, all individuals in a position to influence or control content development are required by NEI to disclose any financial relationships or apparent conflicts of interest. Although potential conflicts of interest are identified and resolved prior to the activity, it remains for the audience to determine whether outside interests reflect a possible bias in either the exposition or the conclusions presented.

These materials have been peer-reviewed to ensure the scientific accuracy and medical relevance of information presented and its independence from commercial bias. The Neuroscience Education Institute takes responsibility for the content, quality, and scientific integrity of this CME activity.

Individual Disclosure Statements
Authors
Meghan M. Grady
Director, Content Development, Neuroscience Education Institute, Carlsbad, CA
No other financial relationships to disclose.

Stephen M. Stahl, MD, PhD
Adjunct Professor, Department of Psychiatry, University of California, San Diego School of Medicine
Grant/Research: AstraZeneca, CeNeRx BioPharma, Forest, Genomind, Lilly, Merck, Neuronetics, Pamlab, Pfizer, Roche, Sunovion, Servier, Shire, Torrent, Trovis
Consultant/Advisor: Abbott, ACADIA, AstraZeneca, AVANIR, BioMarin, Bristol-Myers Squibb, CeNeRx BioPharma, Dey (Mylan Specialty), Forest, Genomind, GlaxoSmithKline, Johnson & Johnson, Lilly, Lundbeck, Merck, Neuronetics, Novartis, Noven, Ono, Orexigen, Otsuka America, Pamlab, Pfizer, RCT LOGIC, Rexahn, Roche, Servier, Shire, Sunovion, Trius, Trovis, Valeant
Speakers Bureau: Arbor Scientia, AstraZeneca, Forest, Johnson & Johnson, Lilly, Merck, Pfizer, Servier, Sunovion
Board Member: Genomind

Peer Reviewer
William M. Sauvé, MD
Clinical Director, Military Program, Poplar Springs Hospital, Petersburg, VA
Consultant/Advisor: AVANIR
Speakers Bureau: Pfizer, Sunovion

Design Staff
Nancy Muntner, *Director, Medical Illustrations, Neuroscience Education Institute, Carlsbad, CA*
No other financial relationships to disclose.

Program Development
Rory Daley, MPH, *Associate Director, Program Development, Neuroscience Education Institute, Carlsbad, CA*
No other financial relationships to disclose.

Steve Smith, *President and COO, Neuroscience Education Institute, Carlsbad, CA*
No other financial relationships to disclose.

Disclosed financial relationships with conflicts of interest have been reviewed by the Neuroscience Education Institute CME Advisory Board Chair and resolved. All faculty and planning committee members have attested that their financial relationships, if any, do not affect their ability to present well-balanced, evidence-based content for this activity.

Disclosure of Off-Label Use
This educational activity may include discussion of unlabeled and/or investigational uses of agents that are not currently labeled for such use by the FDA. Please consult the product prescribing information for full disclosure of labeled uses.

Disclaimer
Participants have an implied responsibility to use the newly acquired information from this activity to enhance patient outcomes and their own professional development. The information presented in this educational activity is not meant to serve as a guideline for patient management. Any procedures, medications, or other courses of diagnosis or treatment discussed or suggested in this educational activity should not be used by clinicians without evaluation of their patients' conditions and possible contraindications or dangers in use, review of any applicable manufacturer's product information, and comparison with recommendations of other authorities. Primary references and full prescribing information should be consulted.

Sponsorship Information
This activity is sponsored by the Neuroscience Education Institute.

Support
This activity is supported solely by the sponsor, Neuroscience Education Institute. Neither the Neuroscience Education Institute nor Stephen M. Stahl, MD, PhD, has received any funds or grants in support of this educational activity.

Date of Release/Expiration
Release date: October 1, 2012
CME credit expiration date: September 30, 2015. *If this date has passed, please contact NEI for updated information.*

Stahl's Illustrated | Objectives

- Apply evidence-based screening methods to identify patients who are dependent or at risk of becoming dependent on substances of abuse

- Provide preventive counseling and brief interventions for patients at risk of becoming addicted/dependent

- Apply evidence-based treatment strategies to individuals with substance use disorders

- Include strategies for monitoring improvement and addressing adherence as part of the treatment plan for patients with substance use disorders

- Recognize the clinical, behavioral, and neurobiological links between substance use disorders and other disorders of impulsivity

Stahl's Illustrated | Chapter 1

Substance Use and Addiction: An Overview

From a behavioral perspective, addiction can be conceptualized as an impaired ability to inhibit drug seeking in response to environmental information that should normally suppress the behavior. Neurobiologically, this is linked to alterations in reward and other circuitry that may precede initial drug use (e.g., genetic risk factors) and/or be caused by chronic drug exposure itself.

In this book, we provide the biological background that will enable the reader to understand not only how chronic drug exposure is thought to alter reward circuitry, but also how currently available treatments for various substance use disorders work in the brain. We also review screening, treatment, and general management strategies for patients with addiction to various substances of abuse. In addition, we briefly touch on impulse control disorders that may have neurobiological similarities to drug addiction.

This chapter serves as an introduction to these topics by providing clinical definitions of the various terms used to describe substance use and addiction as well as an understanding of the behavioral progression from occasional, impulsive drug use to compulsive use and addiction.

Substance Use Terms

Misuse	Use of a medication other than as directed, whether willful or not
Abuse	Use of a drug/medication for nonmedical purposes (e.g., getting high)
Aberrant Behavior	Medication-related behavior that departs from adherence to the prescription plan
Addiction	Chronic neurobiological disease characterized by impaired control over drug use, compulsive use, continued use despite harm, and/or craving
Pseudo-addiction	Mimics true addiction, but symptoms resolve with adequate pain relief
Dependence	Pharmacological adaptation characterized by drug class-specific withdrawal
Tolerance	State of adaptation in which exposure to a given dose of a drug induces biological changes that result in the drug's diminished effects over time; often leads to dose escalation

TABLE 1.1. Terms related to drug use, addiction, and dependence have historically been used interchangeably; however, this has the potential to create confusion. In this book, we use the term "addiction" when describing the neurobiology of the disease, whereas we generally state "use disorder" when discussing the clinical characteristics and management. Dependence is reserved for describing physiological dependence.

Substance Use Disorder:
Proposed DSM-V Criteria

Maladaptive pattern of substance use leading to significant impairment/distress
(2 or more of the following within 12 months; 2–3 = moderate, >3=severe)

- Recurrent use leading to failure to fulfill major obligations
- Recurrent use in hazardous situations
- Continued use despite persistent or recurrent social problems caused or exacerbated by effects of substance
- Tolerance
- Withdrawal
- Taken in larger amounts or for longer periods than intended
- Persistent desire or unsuccessful efforts to control, reduce, or stop
- Great deal of time spent obtaining, using, or recovering
- Important activities given up or reduced because of substance use
- Continued use despite knowledge of physical or psychological problem likely caused or exacerbated by substance
- Craving or urge to use substance

FIGURE 1.1. Though not finalized yet, the proposed criteria for a substance use disorder in the fifth edition of the *Diagnostic and Statistical Manual of Mental Disorders* (DSM) integrate criteria for abuse and dependence, with the term dependence now limited to physiological dependence (i.e., evidence of tolerance and/or withdrawal). The criteria are the same regardless of the particular substance being used. Separate criteria are still projected to exist for substance-induced intoxication, delirium, and withdrawal.

The Addiction Cycle

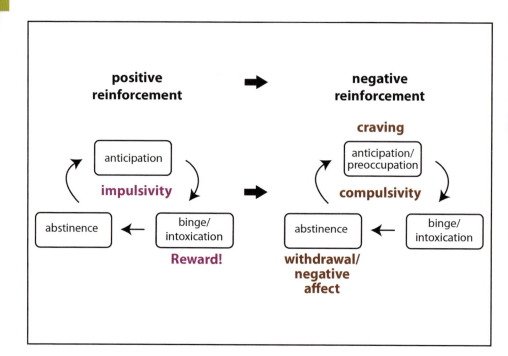

FIGURE 1.2. Addiction can be understood both as a progression from positive to negative reinforcement and as a progression from an impulsive to a compulsive disorder. That is, with initial drug exposure (left), an individual will experience pleasure/reward. This experience "teaches" the brain to anticipate reward on subsequent exposure to the drug. When the drug is taken, pleasure/reward will again be experienced, although this may be followed later by regret.

For most individuals, occasional and controlled drug use remains an impulsive choice driven by positive reinforcement from the drug's rewarding effects. However, for those with risk factors for addiction or excessive drug exposure (see Figure 1.3), this occasional drug use causes neurobiological changes that lead to the development of drug craving, reduced reward on drug exposure, and withdrawal/negative affect state during abstinence (right). Thus, drug addiction can be conceptualized as a compulsive disorder driven by negative reinforcement, wherein the withdrawal symptoms and negative affect during abstinence lead to craving and preoccupation with the drug, with drug use providing relief from these symptoms.

Risk Factors for Addiction

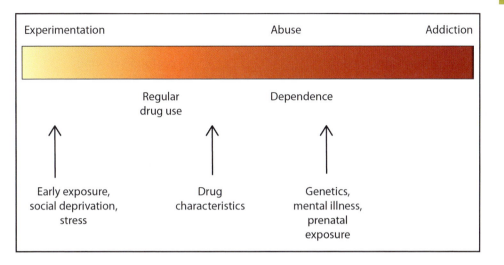

FIGURE 1.3. The risk for developing addiction is affected by multiple factors, including environment, characteristics of the particular drug, and genetics. Environmental risk factors include prenatal exposure, early exposure (e.g., due to parental use in the home or peer use during adolescence), early use, early social deprivation, and psychological stress. The presence of mental illness is also a risk factor for addiction. Drug characteristics include the specific drug used as well as the method of administration (which affects the rate of uptake).

Genetics are also known to affect the vulnerability to addiction; however, there is no single gene linked to addiction. Instead, the data to date suggest that genetic contributions to addiction are the result of the interaction of numerous genetic factors, much like with other psychiatric disorders. It is also possible that epigenetic mechanisms (i.e., changes in gene expression rather than in the genes themselves) contribute to the risk for addiction. For example, early life experiences (e.g., prenatal or early life stress) can cause changes in gene expression that can alter the brain's circuitry and thus increase the risk for the development of addiction.

In general, the risk for the initiation of drug use is associated more with psychosocial factors, whereas the risk for progression to addiction is associated more with neurobiological factors.

Patterns of Addiction by Drug

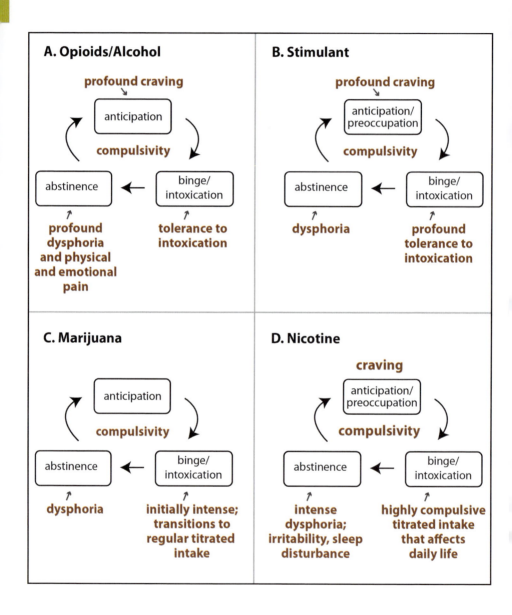

Patterns of Addiction by Drug (cont'd)

FIGURE 1.4. The addiction cycle is the same for all drugs of abuse; however, both the risk of developing addiction and the specific pattern of addiction-related symptoms can vary depending on the particular substance.

(A) Opioids and alcohol initially cause intense intoxication; however, with chronic use, profound tolerance occurs (though some intoxication does remain). This generally results in the escalation of use. Abstinence from opioids/alcohol can lead to serious withdrawal with profound dysphoria and physical and emotional pain.

(B) Stimulants can also cause intense intoxication and binging upon initial use, but, as with opioids/alcohol, profound tolerance to intoxication occurs with chronic use. Preoccupation and craving is generally profound with stimulant addiction. Withdrawal is generally not as intense as with some other substances, although dysphoria can occur.

(C) Marijuana use typically begins with an intense binge/intoxication stage that transitions to regular titrated intake. Dysphoria can occur during abstinence, but craving is not usually profound.

(D) The pattern of nicotine use is generally highly compulsive and titrated, affecting one's schedule of daily activities; however, there is not generally much intoxication. Abstinence can lead to intense dysphoria, irritability, sleep disturbance, and craving.

Clinical Considerations

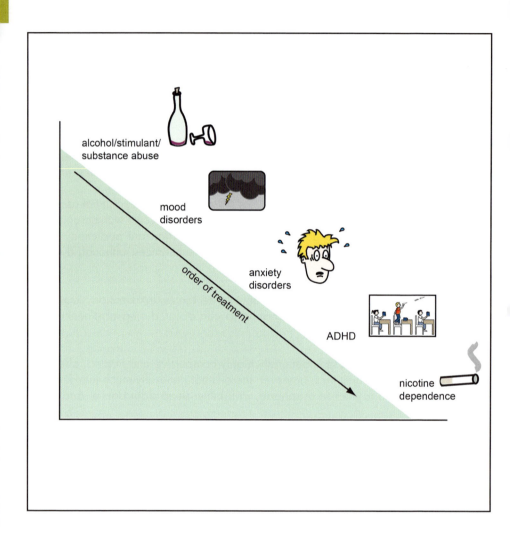

Clinical Considerations (cont'd)

FIGURE 1.5. It is common for individuals with a substance use disorder to use more than one substance. This can complicate the management of patients; unfortunately, there is limited research regarding the treatment of patients who use multiple substances.

Individuals with substance use disorders also have an increased risk of suicide, aggressive behavior (see Figures 10.5 and 10.6), and comorbid psychiatric disorders.

When psychiatric illness and substance use occur comorbidly, it is generally necessary to treat both disorders; in other words, successful treatment of the psychiatric disorder cannot be assumed to resolve the substance use problem. Research and expert clinical opinion support the integrated treatment of both substance use and psychiatric illness. However, depending on the severity of individual disorders, patients may sometimes do better if treatment is sequential rather than simultaneous. In some cases (e.g., major depression), this may mean that the substance use disorder is better treated first, so that one can differentiate between substance-induced symptoms and other symptoms. In many cases, however, it may be better to treat the psychiatric illness first, particularly if symptoms are severe. In general, adherence to psychiatric medication is better if the substance use disorder is treated first. This decision generally needs to be made on a patient-by-patient basis.

The presence of a substance use disorder does not generally affect the medication selection for a psychiatric disorder, although there are some exceptions to this. For example, one would not generally prescribe a benzodiazepine for anxiety for a patient who is actively abusing alcohol; agents that prolong the QTc interval should be avoided in patients abusing stimulants; some medications (olanzapine, clozapine, and others) are metabolized by CYP450 1A2, which is induced by cigarette smoking; and tricyclic antidepressants may be of greater concern in patients with SUDs because of the risk of seizures.

Stahl's Illustrated | Chapter 2

The Neurobiology of Reward and Drug Addiction

The goal of neurobiological drug abuse research is to identify the mechanisms that mediate the progression from occasional and impulsive drug use to compulsive drug use, as well as how these mechanisms contribute to the high risk for relapse even after prolonged abstinence. It is known that chronic drug use affects not only dopamine and the reward circuit, but also other neurotransmitters and circuits involved in memory, motivation, executive function, and stress. Thus, the mechanisms by which addiction may develop are widespread, and although research is plentiful and rapidly expanding, many unanswered questions still remain.

This chapter covers what is best understood about the neurobiology of the reward system and the acute effects of drug exposure; chronic drug exposure and the progression to addiction; and the neurobiology of tolerance, withdrawal, and the risk for relapse.

Dopamine is Central to Reward

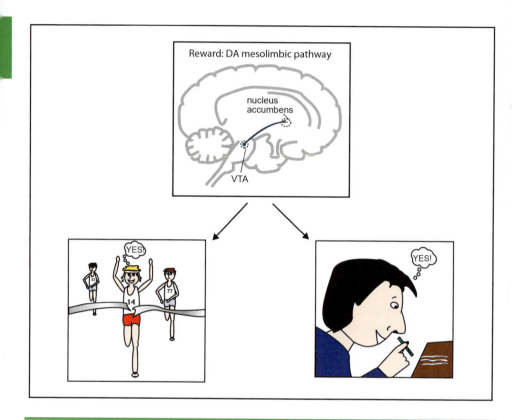

FIGURE 2.1. Dopamine (DA) has long been recognized as a major player in the regulation of reinforcement and reward. Specifically, the mesolimbic pathway from the ventral tegmental area (VTA) to the nucleus accumbens seems to be crucial for reward. Naturally rewarding activities, such as achieving major accomplishments or enjoying a good meal, can cause fast and large increases in DA in the mesolimbic pathway. Drugs of abuse also cause DA release in the mesolimbic pathway, although the mechanisms by which they achieve this can vary (see Table 2.1). In fact, drugs of abuse can often increase dopamine in a manner that is more explosive and pleasurable than that which occurs naturally. Unfortunately, unlike a natural high, the activation caused by drugs of abuse can eventually cause changes in reward circuitry that are associated with a vicious cycle of drug preoccupation, craving, addiction, dependence, and withdrawal.

Dopamine Pathways Involved in Reward

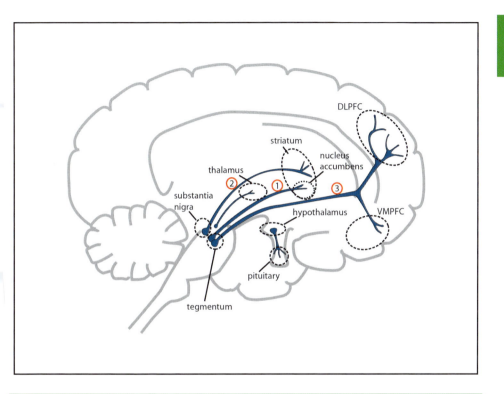

FIGURE 2.2. Although the mesolimbic dopamine pathway (1) is central to reward, other dopaminergic pathways are involved as well—notably, the nigrostriatal pathway (2, substantia nigra to dorsal striatum) and the mesocortical pathway [3, VTA to ventromedial prefrontal cortex (VMFC) and dorsolateral prefrontal cortex (DLPFC)].

Dopamine and Drugs of Abuse

Drug	Target	Mechanism of DA Increase
Stimulants	Dopamine transporter (DAT)	Blocks DAT on DA neurons projecting from VTA to NAc (cocaine) or releases DA from DA terminals (methamphetamine, amphetamine)
Opioids	Mu-opioid receptor (MOR)	Disinhibits VTA DA neurons by inhibiting GABA interneurons that contain MOR in the VTA or directly activates NAc neurons that contain MOR
Nicotine	Nicotine receptors (mainly alpha 4 beta 2)	Directly activates VTA DA neurons via stimulation at their nicotine receptors and indirectly activates them by stimulating the nicotine receptors in glutamatergic terminals to VTA DA neurons
Alcohol and inhalants	Multiple, including GABA and glutamate receptors	Facilitates GABAergic neurotransmission, which may disinhibit VTA DA neurons from GABA interneurons or may inhibit glutamate terminals that regulate DA release in NAc
Cannabinoids	Cannabinoid CB1	Regulates DA signaling through CB1 receptors in NAc neurons and in GABA and glutamate terminals to NAc

DA: dopamine. VTA: ventral tegmental area. NAc: nucleus accumbens. GABA: gamma aminobutyric acid.

TABLE 2.1. All drugs of abuse increase dopamine in the nucleus accumbens, either directly or indirectly.

Dopamine, Pharmacokinetics, and Reinforcing Effects

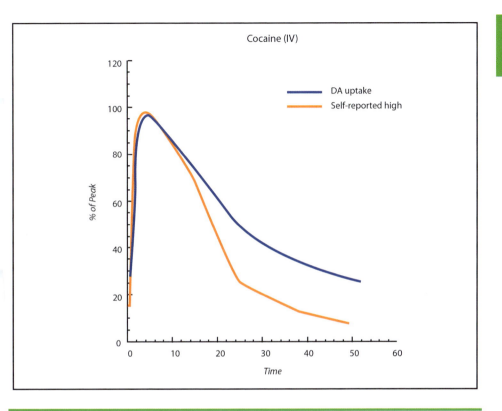

FIGURE 2.3. As already discussed, acute drug use causes DA release in the striatum. However, the reinforcing effects of the drug are largely determined not only by the presence of DA, but also by the rate at which DA increases in the brain, which in turn is dictated by the speed at which the drug enters and leaves the brain. This is likely because abrupt and large increases in DA (such as those caused by drugs of abuse) mimic the phasic DA firing associated with conveying information about reward and saliency.

The rate of drug uptake is subject to the route of administration, with intravenous administration and inhalation producing the fastest drug uptake, followed by snorting. In addition, different drugs of abuse have different "reward values" (i.e., different rates at which they increase DA) based on their individual mechanisms of action.

Neurotransmitter Regulation of Mesolimbic Reward

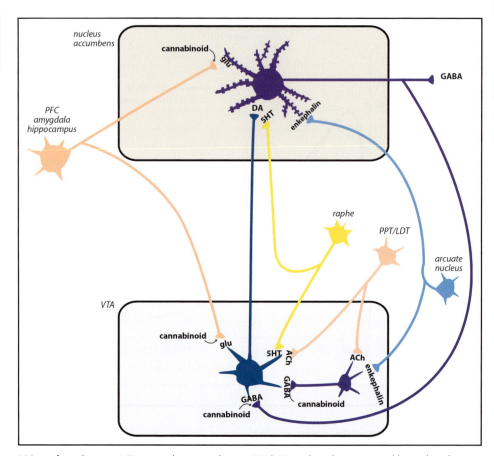

PFC: prefrontal cortex. VTA: ventral tegmental area. PPT/LDT: pedunculopontine and laterodorsal tegmental nucleus. ACh: acetylcholine. Glu: glutamate. DA: dopamine. 5HT: serotonin. GABA: gamma aminobutyric acid.

FIGURE 2.4. Although dopamine is a final common pathway of reward, many other neurotransmitters are involved and in some cases critical, as illustrated here. Of particular importance is the opioid system, which mediates hedonic evaluation of natural rewards. This system also seems to play a role in drug reinforcement for numerous substances. Knockout of the mu opioid receptor in mice not only eliminates reinforcement to opioids (measured by conditioned place preference or self-administration), but also reduces alcohol consumption, reward associated with nicotine, and reward associated with cannabinoids.

Substrates for the Reinforcing Effects of Drugs of Abuse

		Stimulant	Opioid	Alcohol	Nicotine	THC
Neurotransmitter	DA	X	X	X	X	X
	GABA			X	X	X
	Opioid		X	X	X	X
	CB		X	X		X
	ACh				X	
Site of Action	NA	X	X	X	X	X
	AMYG	X		X	X	
	VTA		X	X	X	X

DA: dopamine. GABA: gamma aminobutyric acid. CB: endocannabinoid. ACh: nicotinic acetylcholine. NA: nucleus accumbens. AMYG: amygdala. VTA: ventral tegmental area. THC: delta-9-tetrahydrocannabinol.

TABLE 2.2. The neurotransmitters and sites of action for major drugs of abuse.

The Reactive Reward System

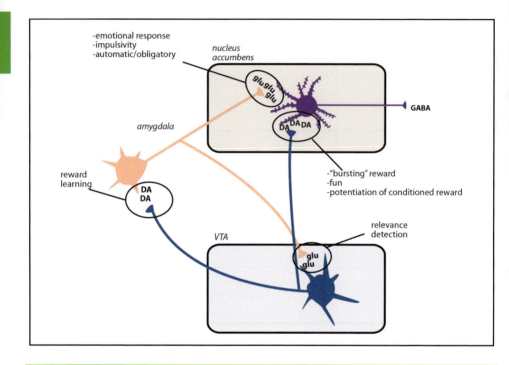

FIGURE 2.5. One way to conceptualize the reward system is to consider it as made up of two complementary parts: one that is reactive and one that is reflective. The reactive reward system, shown here, is a "bottom up" system that signals the immediate prospect of either pleasure or pain and provides motivation and behavioral drive either to achieve that pleasure or avoid that pain. For example, internal cues such as craving and withdrawal cause the reactive reward system to trigger drug-seeking behavior. The reactive reward system consists of the VTA, which is the site of DA cell bodies; the nucleus accumbens, where DA neurons project; and the amygdala, which connects to both the VTA and the nucleus accumbens. Rewarding input to the nucleus accumbens is due to bursts of DA release (i.e., phasic DA firing). Connections of dopaminergic neurons to the amygdala are involved in reward learning (such as the memory of pleasure associated with drug abuse), while connections of the amygdala back to the VTA communicate whether anything relevant to a previously experienced pleasure has been detected. Connections of the amygdala to the nucleus accumbens communicate that emotions have been triggered by internal or external cues and signal an impulsive, almost reflexive response to be taken.

The Reflective Reward System

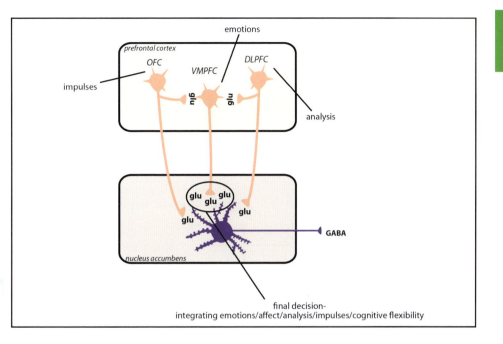

FIGURE 2.6. Stimulatory input from the "bottom up" reactive reward system (Figure 2.5) is regulated by the "top down" reflective reward system, which consists of projections from the prefrontal cortex to the nucleus accumbens. Projections from the orbitofrontal cortex (OFC) are involved in regulating impulses, projections from the dorsolateral prefrontal cortex (DLPFC) are involved in analyzing situations and regulating whether an action takes place, and projections from the ventromedial prefrontal cortex (VMPFC) are involved in regulating emotions. In addition, the insula (not pictured) is reciprocally connected to the amygdala, the VMPFC, and the ventral striatum and is necessary (along with the VMPFC) for emotional decision-making. When all the inputs are integrated, the final output is either to stop the action that the reactive reward system is triggering (e.g., drug seeking) or to let it happen.

The reflective reward system is built and maintained over time based on various influences, including neurodevelopment, genetics, peer pressure, the learning of social rules, and the learning of the benefits of suppressing current pleasure for more valuable future gain. When fully developed and functioning properly, the reflective reward system can shape the final output of the reward system into long-term beneficial goal-directed behaviors.

Temptation vs. Willpower

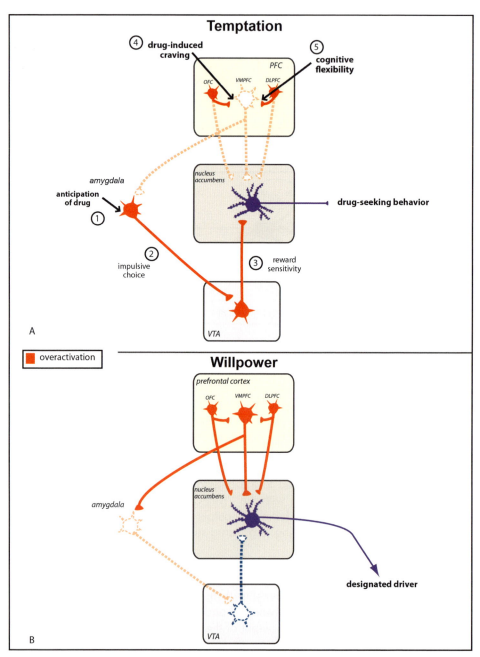

Temptation vs. Willpower (cont'd)

FIGURE 2.7. Temptation may be seen as "bottom up" demand from the reactive reward system, while willpower is a result of "top down" decision-making by the reflective reward system.

(A) When drug anticipation occurs, (1) this signals an impulsive choice (2) to the VTA to release dopamine in the nucleus accumbens (3), which in turn produces output to engage in behavior that leads to drug ingestion again. In the prefrontal cortex, the orbitofrontal cortex signals drug-induced cravings and thus supports the "vote" for drug ingestion (4). The dorsolateral prefrontal cortex interprets the various signals and, showing cognitive flexibility, decides whether to take the action of drug ingestion (5).

(B) If the reflective reward system (prefrontal circuitry) is activated (shown here by the prefrontal neurons turning red), this can prevent impulses (temptation) from being expressed as behavior.

Turning Reward Into Goal-Directed Behavior

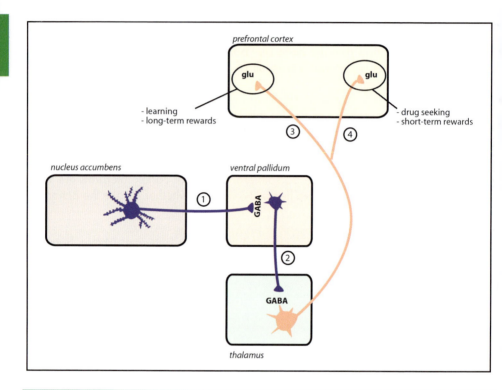

FIGURE 2.8. As shown in Figure 2.6, the reflective reward system is made up of projections from the prefrontal cortex to the striatum (specifically, the nucleus accumbens). Output of the reward system (i.e., turning reward into goal-directed behavior), in turn occurs by means of GABA-ergic neurons projecting from the nucleus accumbens to another part of the striatum, the ventral pallidum (1), from which GABA-ergic neurons project to the thalamus (2). Connections from the thalamus project back up to the prefrontal cortex, where behaviors are implemented [e.g., learning and activities involved in long-term reward (3) or drug-seeking behavior leading to short-term reward (4)].

Conditioning to Reward Cues:
DA

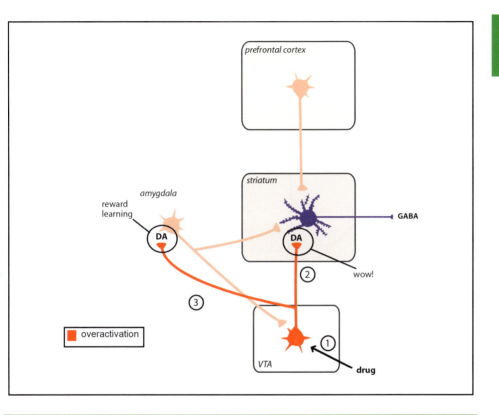

FIGURE 2.9. What mediates the transition from occasional, controlled drug use to drug craving and compulsive drug seeking and use?

One of the earlier neuroadaptations following drug exposure is the process of conditioning. Drug exposure (1) causes an increase in DA in the dorsal striatum (depicted by red color of neurons) and a corresponding increase in pleasure (2). As a result, the amygdala "learns" that this is a rewarding experience (3).

Compulsive Use/Addiction

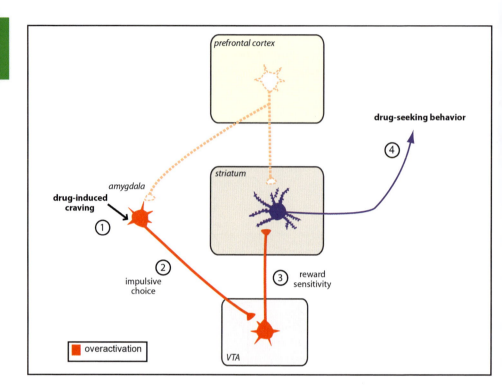

Compulsive Use/Addiction (cont'd)

FIGURE 2.10. Over time, increases in DA in the dorsal striatum are triggered by neutral stimuli associated with the drug reinforcer. This occurs in anticipation of the reward and is associated with drug craving and drug seeking. Thus, when cues are encountered, the amygdala signals to DA neurons in the VTA that something good is coming; it may even signal relief from drug craving (1 and 2). This leads to DA release in the striatum (3), which triggers GABA-ergic input to the thalamus and thalamic input to the prefrontal cortex. As long as the reflective reward system is not activated, this leads to action such as drug-seeking behavior (4).

The dorsal striatum is associated with habit learning, suggesting that the conditioned response triggered by DA results in habits that lead to compulsive drug use. In fact, with repeated drug use, the conditioned drug cues (formally neutral stimuli) can stimulate greater increases in DA than the drug of abuse itself.

In addicted individuals, exposure to drug or drug cues is associated with increased metabolism in the ventral anterior cingulate cortex, the medial orbitofrontal cortex (impulsivity), and the dorsal striatum. This increase in metabolism is associated with drug craving and appears to occur only in drug-addicted individuals. Thus, it appears to be associated specifically with addiction and the corresponding enhanced desire/craving for drug, rather than with drug exposure in general. Additionally, drug-addicted individuals have reduced dopamine 2 receptors in the striatum, which is associated with decreased metabolism in the dorsolateral prefrontal cortex (analysis).

Loss of Control Over Drug Use:
The Prefrontal Cortex and Glutamate

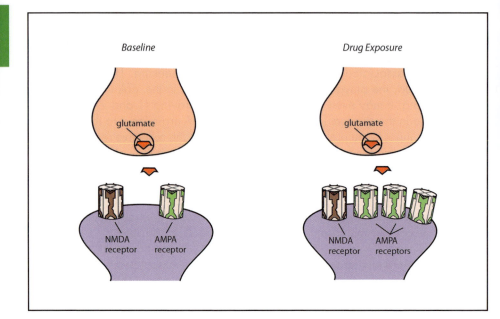

Loss of Control Over Drug Use:
The Prefrontal Cortex and Glutamate (cont'd)

FIGURE 2.11. The reinforcement of drug seeking is linked to not only dopaminergic activation in the reactive reward system but also glutamatergic dysfunction in the reflective reward system. Specifically, there seems to be a disruption in function with glutamatergic projections from the prefrontal cortex to the VTA and the nucleus accumbens.

Glutamate activity heavily modulates synaptic plasticity and therefore learning. Thus, glutamatergic dysfunction and the development of addiction can be viewed as a process of pathological learning and memory. This is specifically modulated through changes in the ratio of N-methyl-d-aspartate (NMDA) and alpha amino-3-hydroxy-5-methyl-4-isoxazolepropionic acid (AMPA) receptors in the VTA, receptors that are known to be involved in long-term potentiation (LTP). That is, stimulation of NMDA receptors leads to calcium influx, which in turn leads to AMPA receptor upregulation and a corresponding increase in the AMPA/NMDA receptor ratio. This reflects an increase in synaptic strength, which should facilitate learning associated with the drug exposure.

The administration of multiple drugs of abuse (cocaine, amphetamine, nicotine, morphine, and ethanol) can elicit LTP at excitatory synapses on VTA DA neurons, while pretreatment with an NMDA antagonist can block this effect. NMDA receptor blockade in the VTA also prevents behavioral effects associated with addiction (e.g., conditioned place preference and behavioral sensitization in animal models). Stress, a common trigger of relapse, has also been shown to elicit LTP by increasing the AMPA/NMDA receptor ratio, albeit through different mechanisms.

The effects on the AMPA/NMDA receptor ratio are the same after repeated drug exposure as they are after single drug exposure. Therefore, drug-induced LTP at excitatory synapses on VTA DA neurons likely contributes to the early changes in neural circuitry that are associated with the development of addiction, whereas adaptations in downstream circuitry may be more important for longer-lasting behavioral changes.

The Addiction Cycle and Recruitment of the Brain Stress System

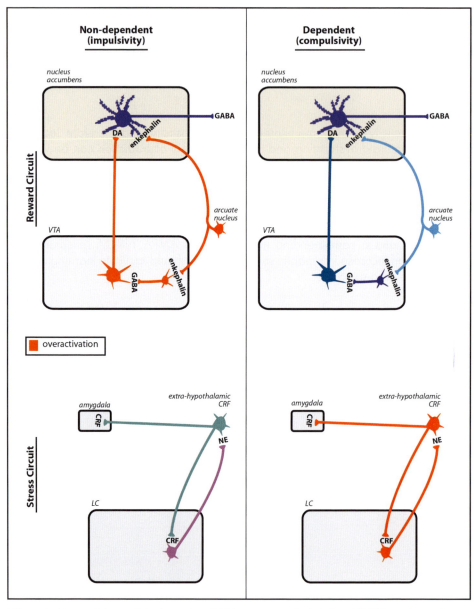

VTA: ventral tegmental area. DA: dopamine. GABA: gamma aminobutyric acid. CRF: corticotropin releasing factor. LC: locus coeruleus. NE: norepinephrine.

The Addiction Cycle and Recruitment of the Brain Stress System (cont'd)

FIGURE 2.12. The progression from occasional, impulsive drug use to compulsive use and addiction involves both the dysregulation of reward circuits and the recruitment of brain/hormonal stress responses. The stress circuit primarily implicated in addiction consists of the extended amygdala in the basal forebrain and the extrahypothalamic corticotropin releasing factor (CRF) system.

With initial drug use (left), the reward system is activated (indicated by the red color of the neurons) and the stress system is recruited to compensate for activity in the reward circuitry (normal activation indicated by the baseline color of the neurons). With chronic drug use (right), the reward circuitry is still activated, but less so (indicated by the baseline color of the neurons), whereas activation of the stress system is more pronounced (indicated by the red color of the neurons).

Development of Tolerance and Acute Withdrawal:
Neurotransmitter Changes

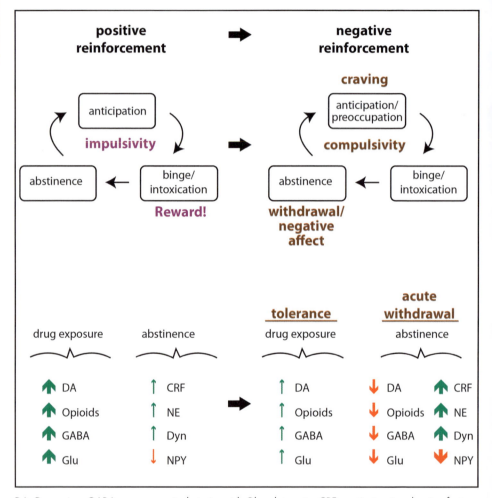

DA: Dopamine. GABA: gamma aminobutyric acid. Glu: glutamate. CRF: corticotropin releasing factor. NE: norepinephrine. Dyn: dynorphin. NPY: neuropeptide Y.

Development of Tolerance and Acute Withdrawal:
Neurotransmitter Changes (cont'd)

FIGURE 2.13. Neurotransmitter changes associated with the dysregulation of reward circuits and the recruitment of brain/hormonal stress responses are shown in Figure 2.13. As these systems become dysregulated, tolerance develops such that the release of "rewarding" neurotransmitters is reduced in response to drug exposure.

During acute withdrawal, there is a decrease in mesolimbic DA activity, reflected in part by a decrease in D2 receptors. There is also decreased activity of opioids, GABA, and glutamate in the nucleus accumbens and the amygdala. In addition, there is recruitment and activation of neurotransmitter systems involved in stress and anxiety, including activation of CRF in the extended amygdala (including the central amygdala), activation of dynorphin (Dyn), activation of norepinephrine (NE), and reduced activity of neuropeptide Y (NPY).

These changes generally occur with all drugs of abuse; however, the overall mechanism of acute withdrawal is likely drug specific, reflecting the adaptations in the molecular targets of the specific drug. For some drugs of abuse (e.g., opioids, alcohol, and sedative hypnotics), acute and intense physical withdrawal occurs and can even be fatal if not properly managed. The management techniques for withdrawal syndromes associated with drugs of abuse are covered in their respective chapters.

Motivational Withdrawal Syndrome

Symptom	Neurotransmitter
Dysphoria	↓ Dopamine ↓ Serotonin ↑ Dynorphin
Anxiety; panic attacks	↓ GABA
Antistress	↓ Neuropeptide Y
Stress	↑ Corticotropin releasing factor ↑ Norepinephrine

TABLE 2.3. Discontinuation of all drugs of abuse can lead to motivational withdrawal syndrome, which is characterized by dysphoria, irritability, emotional distress, and sleep disturbances. The neurotransmitters involved in different symptoms associated with motivational withdrawal syndrome are shown here.

Relapse

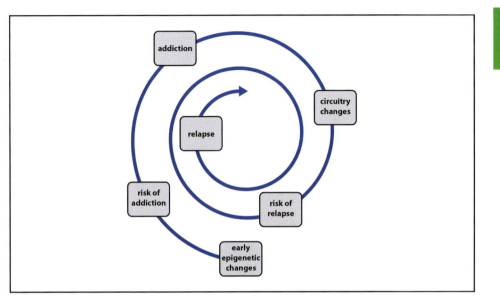

FIGURE 2.14. It may be that chronic drug exposure causes long-term or even permanent changes in gene expression (i.e., epigenetic changes) that in turn lead to long-term or permanent changes in brain circuitry; this would explain the substantial risk for relapse seen with addiction to many drugs of abuse.

In fact, as shown in Figure 1.3, it is even possible that early life experiences (e.g., prenatal or early life stress) can cause changes in gene expression that alter the brain's circuitry and thus increase the risk for the development of addiction in the first place. Those changes would therefore not only persist for an individual who has recovered from addiction, but may also be compounded by additional circuitry changes that occur due to epigenetic mechanisms related to their previous chronic drug use.

Specific neurobiological changes that have been identified in animal studies of stress-induced relapse include an increase in CRF, glucocorticoids, and NE—in other words, persistence of the dysregulation associated with the negative affect state. Animal models of drug-induced relapse/reinstatement implicate the medial prefrontal cortex/nucleus accumbens/glutamatergic circuit that is modulated by DA in the frontal cortex, as well as glutamatergic projections from the basolateral amygdala to the nucleus accumbens.

Stahl's Illustrated | Chapter 3

Alcohol

Alcohol use disorder, like other substance use disorders, is a neurobiological illness in which the normal reward circuitry is changed due to repetitive use of the drug. Knowing the pharmacology of alcohol is therefore important for understanding how addiction and dependence to alcohol take place as well as how they can be treated. This chapter reviews the neurobiological effects of alcohol as well as management strategies for alcohol use disorder, from screening and diagnosis to treatment selection and monitoring.

Actions of Alcohol in the VTA

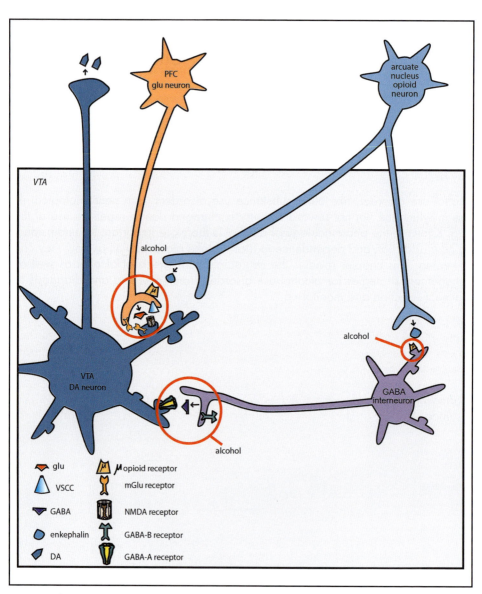

Actions of Alcohol in the VTA (cont'd)

FIGURE 3.1. Although the pharmacology of alcohol is not well characterized, it is generally accepted to act by enhancing inhibitory neurotransmission at GABA synapses while also reducing excitatory neurotransmission at glutamate synapses. Alcohol's euphoric and reinforcing effects may also be related to direct or indirect actions at opioid and cannabinoid synapses and receptors.

In the VTA, alcohol acts at presynaptic metabotropic glutamate (mGlu) receptors and presynaptic voltage-sensitive calcium channels to inhibit glutamate release. Alcohol may also have direct or indirect effects on reducing the actions of glutamate at postsynaptic NMDA receptors and postsynaptic mGlu receptors.

Alcohol enhances GABA release by blocking presynaptic GABA-B receptors. It also acts at postsynaptic GABA-A receptors, particularly those of the delta subtype, which are responsive to neurosteroid modulation but not to benzodiazepines.

Alcohol also has actions at opioid receptors. Opioid neurons, which originate in the arcuate nucleus and project to the VTA, synapse with GABA-ergic interneurons and presynaptic nerve terminals of glutamate neurons. Inhibitory actions of opioids at mu opioid receptors there cause disinhibition of dopamine release in the nucleus accumbens. Alcohol either directly acts upon mu receptors or causes the release of endogenous opioids such as enkephalin.

Pharmacological treatments for alcohol use disorder have been developed utilizing this understanding of alcohol's actions and are shown in Figures 3.11 through 3.16.

What is a Standard Drink?

Standard Serving:

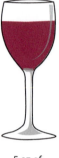 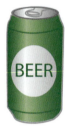

5 oz of table wine   12 oz of beer   1.5 oz of hard alcohol

Typical Restaurant Serving:

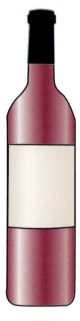 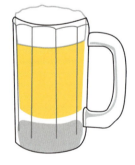 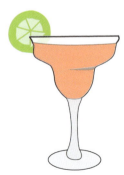

bottle of wine = 5 standard servings   pint of beer = 1.33 standard servings   margarita = 1-3 standard servings

What is a Standard Drink? (cont'd)

FIGURE 3.2. In order to screen effectively for the presence of alcohol abuse or addiction, it is important for both the healthcare provider and the patient to understand what the recommended drinking limits are. This in turn requires that one understand what constitutes a standard drink.

A standard drink contains approximately 14 grams (0.6 fluid ounces, 1.2 tablespoons) of pure alcohol. This translates to approximately 5 ounces of table wine, 12 ounces of beer, or 1.5 ounces of hard alcohol.

To put this in perspective, a typical bottle of wine contains 5 standard drinks (approximately 25 fluid ounces), a typical can of beer is 1 standard drink (12 ounces), and a typical shot of hard alcohol is also 1 standard drink (1.5 ounces). In restaurants and bars, however, a single "drink" may actually be more than 1 standard drink: a serving of draft beer may be more than 12 ounces (e.g., a pint is 16 fluid ounces), while mixed drinks may contain more than 1 shot of alcohol. Thus, without clarifying, a patient's alcohol intake may easily be underestimated.

Recommended Drinking Limits

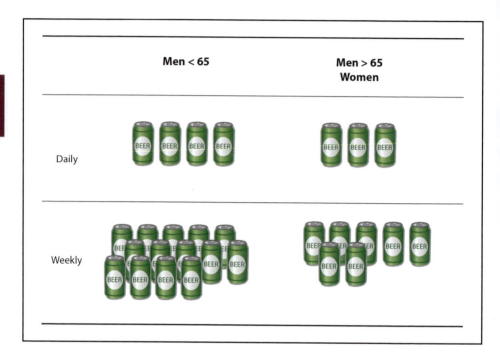

FIGURE 3.3. The recommended drinking limits for men under the age of 65 are no more than 4 drinks in 1 day and no more than 14 drinks in 1 week (National Institute on Alcohol Abuse and Alcoholism, or NIAAA). For men 65 and older and for women, the recommended drinking limits are no more than 3 drinks per day and no more than 7 drinks per week. Amounts in excess of this are considered heavy or at-risk drinking but may not necessarily constitute alcohol use disorder.

Categorizing Drinking Behavior

Abstinent or Low Risk	At Risk	Harmful	Dependent	Chronic Dependent
Drinks less than the NIAAA limits	Drinks more than NIAAA limits 12 or more times per year	Drinks more than NIAAA limits monthly or daily	Drinks 6-10 drinks/day every or nearly every day	Drinks 10 or more drinks/day every or nearly every day
No disability	No disability	Limited disability	Mild to moderate disability	Moderate to severe disability

FIGURE 3.4. Although the objective amount of alcohol consumption is not a part of the diagnostic criteria for alcohol use disorder, it can be useful, in conjunction with degree of disability, for helping to categorize an individual's risk of having or developing alcohol use disorder. Shown here are general guidelines for assessing a patient's risk. These can be combined with the results of screening tools to determine a diagnosis and management strategy.

Screening Methods:
AUDIT

AUDIT Questions	0	1	2	3	4
How often do you have a drink containing alcohol?	Never	Monthly or less	2-4 times a month	2-3 times a week	4 or more times a week
How many drinks containing alcohol do you have on a typical day when you are drinking?	1 or 2	3 or 4	5 or 6	7 to 9	10 or more
How often do you have six or more drinks on one occasion?	Never	Less than monthly	Monthly	Weekly	Daily or almost daily
How often during the last year have that you were not able to stop drinking once you had started?	Never	Less than monthly	Monthly	Weekly	Daily or almost daily
How often during the last year have you failed to do what was normally expected of you because of drinking?	Never	Less than monthly	Monthly	Weekly	Daily or almost daily
How often during the last year have you needed a first drink in the morning to get yourself going after a heavy drinking session?	Never	Less than monthly	Monthly	Weekly	Daily or almost daily
How often during the last year have you had a feeling of guilt or remorse after drinking?	Never	Less than monthly	Monthly	Weekly	Daily or almost daily
How often during the last year have you been unable to remember what happened the night before because of your drinking?	Never	Less than monthly	Monthly	Weekly	Daily or almost daily
Have you or someone else been injured because of your drinking?	No		Yes, but not in the last year		Yes, during the last year
Has a friend, relative, doctor, or other healthcare worker ever been concerned about your drinking or suggested you cut down?	No		Yes, but not in the last year		Yes, during the last year

Screening Methods:
AUDIT (cont'd)

FIGURE 3.5. Ideally, all patients will be screened with respect to their alcohol use with either a self-report questionnaire filled out prior to interview or a simple prescreen question asked at the start of the interview.

There are multiple self-report screening tools available. The AUDIT (Alcohol Use Disorders Identification Test) was developed by the World Health Organization (WHO) and is recommended by the NIAAA. It consists of 10 questions and can typically be completed in about a minute (shown in Figure 3.5). The CAGE Questionnaire consists of 4 questions and is used in military settings. Other assessments include the Paddington Alcohol Test (PAT) and the Rapid Alcohol Problems Screen (RAPS4).

Instead of using a prescreen self-assessment, it can be beneficial to ask a single question during interview in order to determine if additional follow-up is necessary—namely, "Do you sometimes drink wine, beer, or other alcoholic beverages?" If the answer is yes, one can then ask, "How many times in the past year have you had X (5 for men, 4 for women) or more drinks a day?" Depending on the response, verbally asking additional questions from the AUDIT can help determine the degree of risk and the need for intervention.

A straightforward approach is best when asking these questions; patients are less likely to feel defensive if they perceive the questions as routine and relevant to medical history, much like questions about diet and exercise habits.

Treatment Strategies:
A Function of Drinking Behavior and Willingness to Change, Part 1

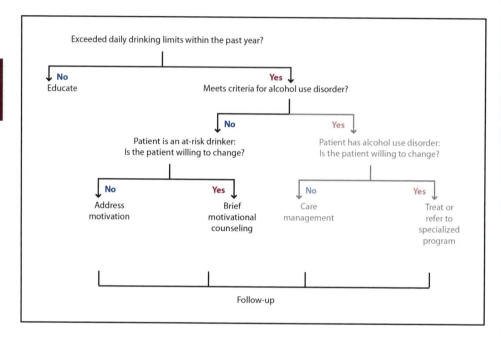

Treatment Strategies:
A Function of Drinking Behavior and Willingness to Change, Part 1 (cont'd)

FIGURE 3.6. Treatment strategies for patients with problem drinking are dependent on both their drinking behaviors and their willingness to change.

For individuals who exceed the recommended drinking limits but do not meet the criteria for alcohol use disorder, it is important to clearly express your concern to them: "You are drinking more than is medically safe, and I strongly recommend that you cut down (or quit)." Relate this recommendation to the patient's concerns and medical findings if possible.

If the patient is willing to make changes to drinking habits, work with him or her to set a goal (cut down to within the maximum limits or abstain for a period of time), and then agree on a plan for achieving it. Decision points include what specific steps the patient will take (not go to a bar after work, measure all drinks at home, alternate alcoholic and non-alcoholic beverages), how drinking will be tracked (diary, kitchen calendar), how the patient will manage high-risk situations, and who might be willing to help (a spouse or nondrinking friends). Providing educational materials is also useful.

If the patient is not yet willing to change, restate your concern about his or her health, encourage reflection (what are the major barriers to change?), and reaffirm your willingness to help when he or she is ready.

Treatment Strategies:
A Function of Drinking Behavior and Willingness to Change, Part 2

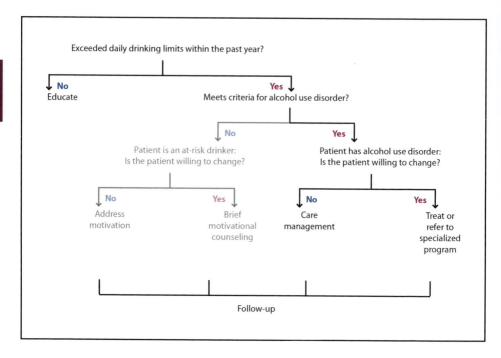

Treatment Strategies:
A Function of Drinking Behavior and Willingness to Change, Part 2 (cont'd)

FIGURE 3.7. For patients with alcohol use disorder, it is also important to state your conclusion and recommendation clearly: "I believe that you have alcohol use disorder. I strongly recommend that you quit drinking, and I'm willing to help." Again, it is useful to relate your recommendation to the patient's concerns and medical findings if possible.

If the patient is willing to make changes, negotiate a drinking goal, with the ideal being abstinence. Treatment can include both a pharmacological option and a psychosocial strategy, such as a mutual help group, motivational enhancement therapy, or cognitive behavioral therapy. Treatment must be coordinated with that for comorbid medical or psychiatric illnesses.

If the patient is not yet willing to change, restate your concern about his or her health, encourage reflection (what are the major barriers to change?), and reaffirm your willingness to help when he or she is ready.

Reduced-Risk Drinking:
An Alternative Outcome, Part 1

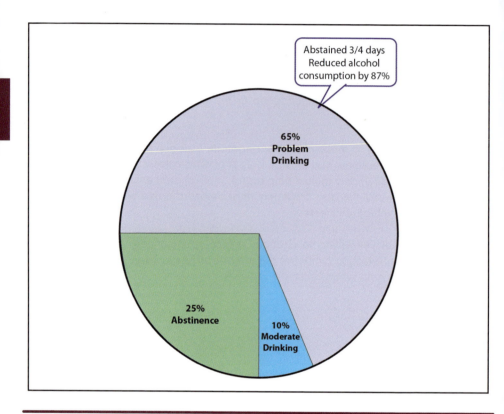

FIGURE 3.8. The ideal goal of treatment for alcohol use disorder is abstinence; however, abstinence does not have to be the only positive outcome of treatment. The majority of patients do not achieve abstinence, and those who do may require multiple tries. Even individuals who do not achieve abstinence may exhibit significant and positive changes in their drinking behavior. Findings from 7 large multisite studies showed that during the year after treatment, 1 in 4 clients remained continuously abstinent on average, and an additional 1 in 10 used alcohol moderately and without problems. During this period, mortality averaged less than 2%. As a group, the remaining clients showed substantial improvement, abstaining on 3 days out of 4 and reducing their overall alcohol consumption by 87% on average. Alcohol-related problems also decreased by 60%.

Reduced-Risk Drinking:
An Alternative Outcome, Part 2

 Potential Goal For:

At-risk drinkers

People with less severe drinking problems

 Contraindicated For:

Conditions that would be exacerbated by alcohol

Use of disulfiram or other agents contraindicated with alcohol

History of failed attempts with reduced-risk drinking

Pregnancy or breastfeeding

History of severe alcohol withdrawal symptoms

FIGURE 3.9. Reduced-risk drinking as a goal is controversial. However, some patients will not agree to abstinence as a goal. For these patients, it can still be beneficial to work with them to reduce their drinking. Reduced-risk drinking may be a better goal for patients with less severe drinking problems, including at-risk drinkers (already shown in Figure 3.6). As with at-risk drinkers, the strategy for achieving reduced-risk drinking for patients with alcohol use disorder involves agreeing on a plan. Give patients a choice in the goal if possible; this allows them to take part in decisions affecting their lives and gives them more responsibility in the outcome. Some sample guidelines for reduced-risk drinking include the "3 As": avoid having more than 1 drink in 1 hour, avoid drinking patterns (same people, same places, same time of day), and avoid drinking to deal with problems.

Contraindications for reduced-risk drinking (as opposed to abstinence) include existing conditions that would be exacerbated by alcohol, the use of disulfiram or other agents contraindicated with alcohol, a history of failed attempts with reduced-risk drinking, pregnancy or breastfeeding, and a history of severe alcohol withdrawal symptoms. For patients who should pursue abstinence but refuse, one may try to have them agree to a trial period of abstinence and a trial period of reduced-risk drinking; it can be beneficial to use a written contract.

Pharmacological Treatment for Alcohol Use Disorder

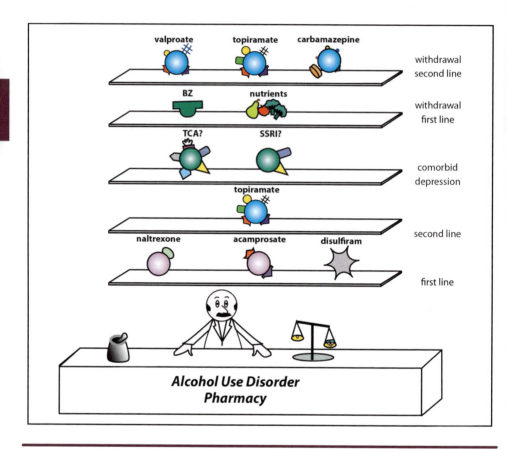

FIGURE 3.10. Pharmacological options to treat alcohol use disorder include naltrexone (available both orally and as an injection), acamprosate, and disulfiram. Topiramate is sometimes used second-line. Selective serotonin reuptake inhibitors (SSRIs) and tricyclic antidepressants (TCAs) have been used in patients with comorbid depression, but with inconsistent results. There are animal studies and preliminary clinical reports of the serotonin 3 antagonist ondansetron to treat alcohol use disorder, but there is no clear evidence that it is effective.

Alcohol withdrawal can be treated pharmacologically with a benzodiazepine (BZ) and the repletion of nutrients. Second-line alternatives to benzodiazepines include carbamazepine, topiramate, and valproate.

Psychosocial Treatment for Alcohol Use Disorder

		CBT	MET	Behavioral therapy	IPT	Family therapy	Self-help/ 12-step
Substance of Abuse	Alcohol	X	X	X		X	X
	Opioid	X		X		X	X
	Nicotine	X	X	X			
	Stimulant	X		X			X
	THC		X	X			

CBT: cognitive behavioral therapy. MET: motivational enhancement therapy. Behavioral therapy: contingency management, community reinforcement, cue exposure and relaxation, aversion therapy. IPT: interpersonal therapy. THC: delta-9-tetrahydrocannabinol.

TABLE 3.1. Psychosocial treatments are an extremely important component of substance use disorder management. Many of the same general strategies are used to treat addiction to/dependence on different substances of abuse. The specific strategies that are commonly used in the treatment of alcohol use disorder are highlighted here. These strategies are explained in more detail in Chapter 9.

Acamprosate

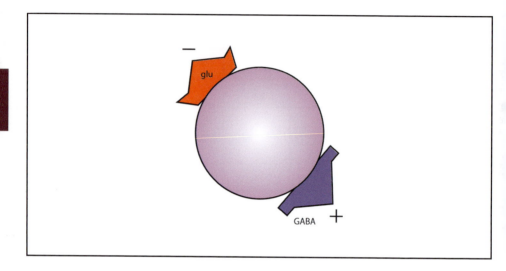

FIGURE 3.11. Acamprosate is a derivative of the amino acid taurine, and like alcohol it reduces excitatory glutamate neurotransmission and enhances inhibitory GABA neurotransmission. In particular, it seems to block mGlu receptors and perhaps also NMDA receptors.

When alcohol is used chronically and then withdrawn, the adaptive changes that it causes in both the glutamate and GABA systems creates a state of glutamate hyperactivity—even excitotoxicity—and GABA deficiency. By blocking glutamate receptors, acamprosate may mitigate glutamate hyperexcitability during alcohol withdrawal and is therefore sometimes called "artificial alcohol."

Acamprosate is intended for use only in patients who have already achieved abstinence.

Acamprosate (Campral):
Tips and Pearls

Dosing and Use

Formulation:
Tablet: 333 mg

Dosage Range:
666 mg 3 times daily (>60 kg)
666 mg 2 times daily (<60 kg)

Approved For:
Maintenance of alcohol abstinence

Pearls

Serves as "artificial alcohol"; may be less effective in situations in which the patient has not yet abstained; patients should continue treatment even if relapse occurs but should disclose any new drinking; dosing schedule may affect adherence; generally well tolerated, with diarrhea as the most common side effect; no known interactions with psychotropic medications (not metabolized by hepatic enzymes; does not inhibit or induce hepatic enzymes)

Side Effects and Safety

Weight Gain

unusual | not unusual | common | problematic

Sedation

unusual | not unusual | common | problematic

 Suicidal ideation and behavior

 Do not use if patient has severe renal impairment

Special Populations

 Safety and efficacy have not been established

 Pregnancy risk category C (some animal studies show adverse effects; no controlled studies in humans)

 Limited available data on patients with cardiac impairment

 For moderate renal impairment, recommended dose is 333 mg 3 times daily; contraindicated in severe impairment

 Dose adjustment not generally necessary for patients with hepatic impairment

FIGURE 3.12. Dosing and safety information for acamprosate.

Naltrexone

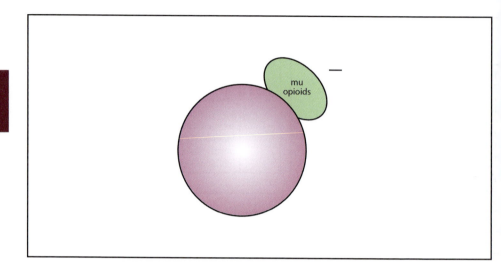

FIGURE 3.13. Naltrexone blocks mu opioid receptors, which theoretically contribute to the euphoria and high associated with drinking. That is, opioid neurons form synapses in the VTA with GABA-ergic interneurons and presynaptic nerve terminals of glutamate neurons. Alcohol either acts directly upon mu opioid receptors or causes the release of endogenous opioids; in either case, the result is increased dopamine release to the nucleus accumbens. It is therefore not surprising that a mu opioid antagonist would block the enjoyment of heavy drinking and potentially increase abstinence.

Naltrexone can be used not only in patients who are abstinent, but also in those who are reducing their drinking. It is available in both oral and monthly injectable formulations.

Naltrexone (Revia, Vivitrol):
Tips and Pearls

Dosing and Use

Formulation:
Tablets: 25 mg, 50 mg, 100 mg
Oral solution: 12 mg/0.6 mL
Intramuscular: 380 mg/vial

Dosage Range:
Oral: 50 mg/day
Injection: 380 mg every 4 weeks

Approved For:
Alcohol dependence
Prevention of relapse to opioid dependence

Side Effects and Safety

Weight Gain

Sedation

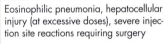
Eosinophilic pneumonia, hepatocellular injury (at excessive doses), severe injection site reactions requiring surgery

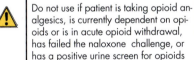
Do not use if patient is taking opioid analgesics, is currently dependent on opioids or is in acute opioid withdrawal, has failed the naloxone challenge, or has a positive urine screen for opioids

Pearls

Can be used in patients who have achieved abstinence, who are trying to achieve abstinence, or who are trying to reduce heavy drinking; less effective in patients who are not abstinent at the time of treatment initiation; adherence is greatly increased with the injectable formulation; side effects include nausea, vomiting, and site reactions (injection); can block the effects of opioid-containing medications; some patients complain of apathy with chronic treatment

Special Populations

Safety and efficacy have not been established

Pregnancy risk category C (some animal studies show adverse effects; no controlled studies in humans)

Limited available data on patients with cardiac impairment

Dose adjustment not generally necessary for mild renal impairment; not studied in moderate to severe impairment

Dose adjustment not generally necessary for mild hepatic impairment; not studied in severe hepatic impairment; contraindicated in acute hepatitis or liver failure

FIGURE 3.14. Dosing and safety information for naltrexone.

Disulfiram

Disulfiram
Antabuse

Dosage Range:
250–500 mg/day, 1-year duration

Approved For:
Maintenance of abstinence

Pearls:
Disulfiram should not be given to a patient in a state of alcohol intoxication or without the patient's full knowledge; the patient should not take disulfiram for at least 12 hours after drinking; a reaction may occur for up to 2 weeks after disulfiram is stopped; the patient should be advised not to consume any food or beverages containing alcohol; the patient should carry an emergency card stating that he or she is taking disulfiram; common side effects include metallic taste, dermatitis, and sedation; potential serious reactions include myocardial infarction, congestive heart failure, respiratory depression, and hepatotoxicity; pregnancy risk category C

Contraindicated in patients taking metronidazole, amprenavir, ritonavir, or sertraline and in those with psychosis or cardiovascular disease; not recommended for patients older than age 60 or for those with severe pulmonary disease, chronic renal failure, diabetes, peripheral neuropathy, seizures, cirrhosis, or portal hypertension

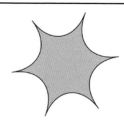

FIGURE 3.15. Alcohol is metabolized to acetaldehyde, which in turn is metabolized by aldehyde dehydrogenase. Disulfiram is an irreversible inhibitor of aldehyde dehydrogenase, thereby blocking this second-stage metabolism. When alcohol is consumed by a patient taking disulfiram, toxic levels of acetaldehyde build up, which leads to flushing, tachycardia, nausea, vomiting, and other symptoms. This aversive experience ideally leads to negative conditioning, in which patients abstain from alcohol in order to avoid the unpleasant effects. Adherence to the medication is of course necessary for this to occur, and not surprisingly, adherence rates can be quite low. In addition, dangerous side effects, including alcohol toxicity, can occur in patients who do not abstain from alcohol while taking disulfiram.

Topiramate

Topiramate
Topamax

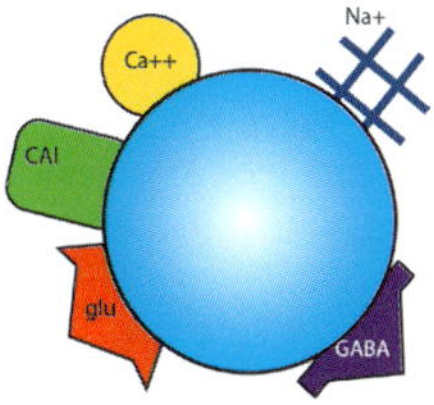

Dosage Range:
Up to 300 mg/day; requires slow upward titration to reduce side effects

Approved For:
Multiple seizure disorders; migraine prophylaxis

Pearls:
May be useful for patients who have achieved abstinence, who are trying to achieve abstinence, or who are trying to reduce heavy drinking; may be useful as an adjunct agent; side effects include sedation, nausea, and weight loss; can cause metabolic acidosis or kidney stones; adverse effects may be dose dependent; lower dose by half for patients with renal impairment; use with caution in patients with hepatic or cardiac impairment and in the elderly; pregnancy risk category C

FIGURE 3.16. Topiramate is an anticonvulsant that inhibits the release of glutamate and potentiates the activity of GABA; these mechanisms also make it a potential option to treat alcohol use disorder. Although not approved for such use, there are some studies demonstrating its effectiveness. Topiramate can be prescribed to patients who have not yet abstained from drinking as either a monotherapy or an adjunct treatment. Topiramate is also a carbonic anhydrase inhibitor and thus may lead to kidney stones, parasthesia, or metabolic acidosis.

Treating Alcohol Withdrawal Syndrome

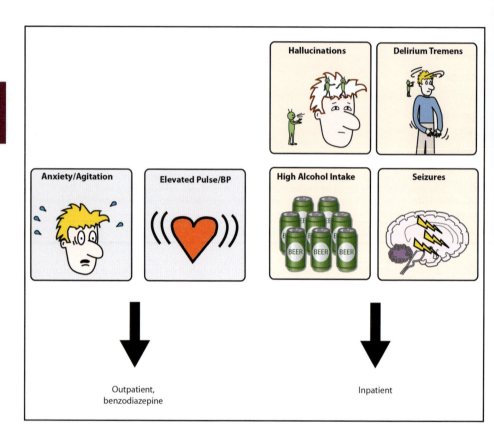

Treating Alcohol Withdrawal Syndrome (cont'd)

FIGURE 3.17. A percentage of individuals who are alcohol dependent will experience alcohol withdrawal syndrome (AWS). Symptoms, which include tremor, elevated pulse rate and blood pressure, sweating, agitation, nervousness, sleeplessness, anxiety, and depression, begin within a few hours of discontinuation and may last a few days to a week. In many cases, AWS resolves without complication and does not require treatment. For some patients, however, intervention is necessary.

For patients with mild to moderate AWS, treatment can be on an outpatient basis and should focus on the relief of immediate symptoms, the prevention of complications, and the initiation of rehabilitation. This may involve supportive care and the repletion of nutrient, fluid, or mineral deficiencies (especially vitamin B). Benzodiazepines are commonly used to reduce anxiety, agitation, and autonomic hyperactivity as well as to reduce the incidence of delirium and seizures. Long-acting benzodiazepines may allow for a smoother course of withdrawal and less frequent dosing, while short-acting benzodiazepines may be preferred for patients with severe liver disorder. Because benzodiazepines have abuse liability and the potential for interaction with alcohol, alternative options may be preferred and include carbamazepine, valproate, or topiramate.

Some patients experience more serious symptoms, such as hallucinations, delirium tremens, psychotic symptoms, and seizures, and require inpatient management. Individuals with extremely high alcohol intake or significant psychiatric symptoms also require inpatient treatment.

Monitoring and Follow-up

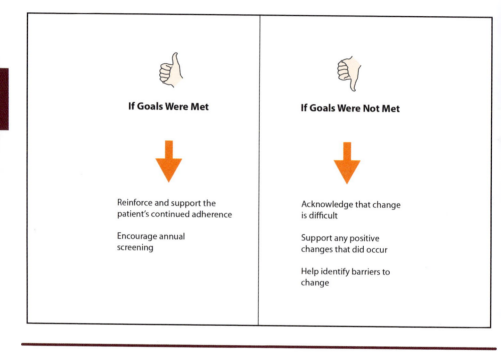

FIGURE 3.18. Monitoring and follow-up are essential components of the treatment strategy for patients with alcohol use disorder or at-risk drinking. At each visit, assess if the patient was able to meet and sustain goals. If so, reinforce and support the patient's continued adherence to recommendations. Encourage the patient to return if they are unable to maintain adherence and rescreen at least annually.

If the patient was not able to maintain or achieve the goal, acknowledge that change is difficult and support any positive changes that did occur while also addressing barriers to reaching the goal. If necessary, renegotiate the goal and plan and make sure that significant others are available to help.

If a patient with at-risk drinking is unable to either cut down or abstain, it may be necessary to reassess the diagnosis.

Stahl's Illustrated | Chapter 4

Opioids

Heroin was first synthesized in the late 1800s and has proven to be one of the most addictive substances known to man. Prescription opioids, including morphine and oxycodone, also have high abuse potential; but until relatively recently, these agents were restricted mainly to palliative care and cancer patients. Now, however, prescription opioid use for the treatment of chronic noncancer pain has gained acceptance and become much more common. Correspondingly, misuse, abuse, and diversion of prescription opioids has increased dramatically and now far exceeds that of heroin. This has substantial consequences; thousands more Americans die each year from unintentional overdose with prescription opioids than from overdose with either heroin or cocaine. Opioid use disorder is therefore a significant public health concern. This chapter reviews the neurobiological effects of opioids as well as screening and management strategies for opioid use disorder.

Actions of Opioids on Reward Circuits

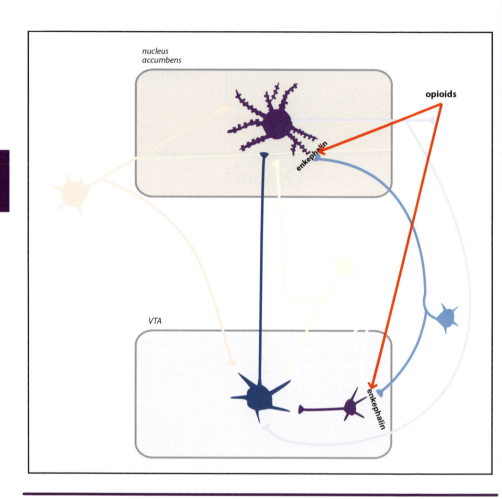

FIGURE 4.1. Neurons originating in the arcuate nucleus project to both the ventral tegmental area (VTA), the site of dopamine cell bodies, and the nucleus accumbens, to which dopaminergic neurons project. Opioid neurons release endogenous opioids (e.g., enkephalin), which mediate the hedonic evaluation of natural rewards and are involved (particularly in the VTA and the nucleus accumbens) in the motivational aspects of dependence and aversive states.

Endogenous Opioid Neurotransmitters

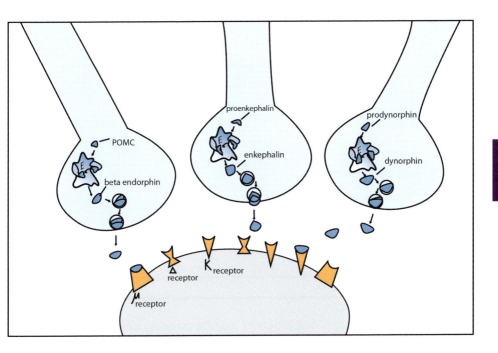

FIGURE 4.2. Endogenous opioids are peptides derived from precursor proteins called POMC (pro-opiomelanocortin), proenkephalin, and prodynorphin. Parts of these precursor proteins are cleaved off to form endorphins, enkephalins, or dynorphins, which are then stored in opioid neurons and released during neurotransmission to mediate reinforcement and pleasure via their actions at a variety of opioid receptors, the most important of which are mu, delta, and kappa.

Mu receptors in the VTA are critically involved in reinforcement and are also involved in drug dependence. Kappa receptors induce dysphoria, counteract mu receptors, and are involved in stress-related drug intake. Delta receptors are involved in emotional control.

Exogenous opioids are also thought to act at mu, delta, and kappa receptors, particularly mu receptors. Specifically, mu and possibly delta receptors in the VTA and the nucleus accumbens mediate the positive reinforcing properties of exogenous opioids.

Screening for Opioid Misuse

Warning Signs	Intoxication	Withdrawal
Vague history	Constricted pupils	Dysphoric mood
Poor rapport	Slurred speech	Nausea/vomiting
Lost/stolen meds	Itching	Muscle aches
Early renewal request	Euphoria or agitation	Runny nose
Urgent calls	Dry mouth	Dilated pupils
Doctor shopping	Drowsiness	Goose bumps
No relief without opioids	Poor judgment	Sweating
Other drug/alcohol abuse		Diarrhea
		Yawning
		Fever
		Insomnia

FIGURE 4.3. Warning signs that a patient may be misusing opioids include vague, inconsistent, or incomplete information in their history; difficulty establishing a rapport; evidence of doctor shopping; reporting lost or stolen medications; early renewal requests; urgent calls or unscheduled visits; no relief with anything except opioids; and evidence of abuse of other drugs or alcohol. Individuals who are acutely intoxicated demonstrate constricted pupils, slurred speech, itching, euphoria or agitation, dry mouth, drowsiness, and impaired judgment. Individuals who are undergoing opioid withdrawal may experience dysphoric mood, nausea or vomiting, muscle aches, runny nose and eyes, dilated pupils, goose bumps, sweating, diarrhea, yawning, fever, and insomnia.

If opioid misuse is suspected, a screening tool may be used for further assessment. There is no single accepted tool. Examples of self-report tools include the Current Opioid Misuse Measure and the Opioid Risk Tool. Examples of comprehensive tools include the Drug Abuse Screening Test, CAGE-AID, and UNCOPE.

Pharmacological Treatment for Opioid Use Disorder

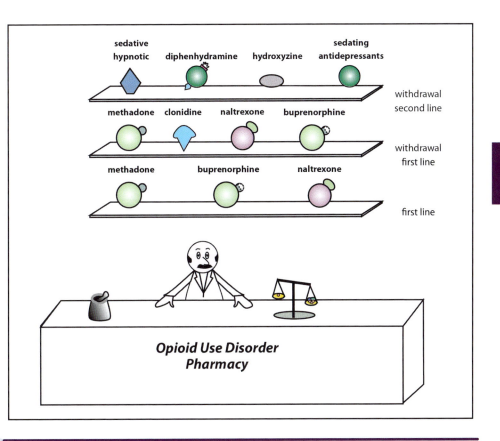

FIGURE 4.4. Pharmacologic options to treat opioid use disorder include methadone (through regulated programs), buprenorphine, and naltrexone. In addition, medications are used specifically to treat opioid withdrawal, including methadone substitution, clonidine, clonidine/naltrexone, and buprenorphine. Other medications that have been used for withdrawal symptom management include sedative hypnotics, anxiolytics, diphenhydramine, hydroxyzine, and sedating antidepressants.

Psychosocial Treatment for Opioid Use Disorder

		CBT	MET	Behavioral therapy	IPT	Family therapy	Self-help/ 12-step
Substance of Abuse	Alcohol	X	X	X		X	X
	Opioid	X		X		X	X
	Nicotine	X	X	X			
	Stimulant	X		X			X
	THC		X	X			

CBT: cognitive behavioral therapy. MET: motivational enhancement therapy. Behavioral therapy: contingency management, community reinforcement, cue exposure and relaxation, aversion therapy. IPT: interpersonal therapy. THC: delta-9-tetrahydrocannabinol.

TABLE 4.1. Psychosocial treatments are an extremely important component of substance use disorder management. Many of the same general strategies are used to treat addiction to/dependence on different substances of abuse. The specific strategies that are commonly used in the treatment of opioid use disorder are highlighted here. These strategies are explained in more detail in Chapter 9.

Treatment Settings

	Inpatient	Outpatient clinic/office	Outpatient opioid treatment program	Drug-free program
Overdose	X	–	–	–
Withdrawal	methadone, buprenorphine*, naltrexone, clonidine	buprenorphine*, naltrexone, clonidine	methadone, buprenorphine	–
Maintenance	–	X	X	X

*requires DEA DATA 2000 waiver

TABLE 4.2. Patients who are dependent on opioids and ready to accept treatment can be managed in different settings, depending on their individual preferences and needs. Inpatient hospitalization is necessary for those who have overdosed and may also be preferred while individuals are undergoing withdrawal (treatment for withdrawal will require outpatient follow-up).

It is also possible to manage patients undergoing withdrawal in an outpatient clinic or office. Clinicians in group or individual practices may provide naltrexone or, if they obtain a DEA DATA 2000 waiver, buprenorphine. Outpatient opioid treatment programs are also an option. These primarily offer methadone, although some may offer buprenorphine.

Individuals who have undergone withdrawal may have ongoing outpatient medication maintenance or may join a drug-free program, which does not provide opioid agonists but may provide naltrexone.

Methadone

Methadone
Dolophine, Methadose

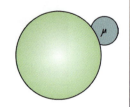

Dosage Range:
Generally 40–100 mg/day

Approved For:
Detoxification treatment of opioid addiction;
maintenance treatment of opioid addiction;
moderate to severe pain not responsive to non-narcotic analgesics

Pearls:
Patients may experience a withdrawal syndrome if methadone is stopped abruptly or administered with an opioid antagonist or partial agonist; common side effects include constipation, sweating, and sexual dysfunction; potential serious reactions include respiratory depression and death from overdose; metabolized primarily by CYP450 3A4, so monitor patients starting or ending a CYP450 3A4 inhibitor or inducer; antiretroviral drugs may increase the clearance of methadone; use caution if administering an agent known to prolong the QT interval or capable of inducing electrolyte disturbances; use caution if the patient is receiving a CNS depressant, particularly a benzodiazepine; use with caution in patients with liver impairment and in those at risk of developing a prolonged QT interval; pregnancy risk category C; contraindicated in patients with respiratory depression, acute bronchial asthma or hypercarbia, or paralytic ileus

Methadone (cont'd)

FIGURE 4.5. Methadone is a mu opioid receptor agonist that blocks the effects of opioids while suppressing the withdrawal symptoms. It is available only through Opioid Treatment Programs (OTPs) that are certified by the Federal Substance Abuse and Mental Health Services Administration (SAMHSA) and registered by the Drug Enforcement Administration (DEA). It is most effective for suppressing use in highly-dependent patients and should be combined with nonpharmacological services (individual/group counseling, urine testing, behavioral treatment).

Methadone is orally active and can be administered once daily. The goal of methadone dosing is to suppress the patient's specific withdrawal symptoms and craving; thus, dosing is very individualized, but generally falls in the 40–100 mg/day range. Specifically, 40–60 mg/day is often sufficient to block opioid withdrawal symptoms, whereas higher doses are usually needed to block craving.

Methadone can be used to treat opioid withdrawal and can also be used as a maintenance treatment. Maintenance treatment with methadone typically lasts 1–2 years but can be longer.

Buprenorphine

Buprenorphine
Subutex, Suboxone (with naloxone)

Dosage Range:
Sublingual: generally 8–32 mg/day
Can be given less often than once daily; double the dose for each additional 24-hour interval

Approved For:
Maintenance treatment of opioid dependence

Pearls:
Patients must be in a mild withdrawal state prior to starting buprenorphine; buprenorphine is available parenterally or sublingually; sublingual formulation can be buprenorphine alone or in combination with naloxone; sublingual formulation must be placed under the tongue and should not be chewed or swallowed; patients may experience a mild withdrawal syndrome if buprenorphine is stopped abruptly; common side effects include oral hypoesthesia, glossodynia, headache, and constipation; potential serious reactions include respiratory depression and death from overdose (less common than with methadone); metabolized by CYP450 3A4, so monitor patients starting or ending a CYP450 3A4 inhibitor or inducer; use caution if the patient is receiving a CNS depressant, particularly a benzodiazepine; use with caution and lower dose in patients with liver impairment; pregnancy risk category C

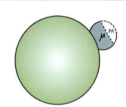

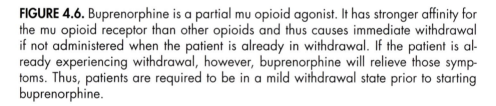

FIGURE 4.6. Buprenorphine is a partial mu opioid agonist. It has stronger affinity for the mu opioid receptor than other opioids and thus causes immediate withdrawal if not administered when the patient is already in withdrawal. If the patient is already experiencing withdrawal, however, buprenorphine will relieve those symptoms. Thus, patients are required to be in a mild withdrawal state prior to starting buprenorphine.

Buprenorphine is considered a "take-home" medication that generally has less stigma and better adherence than methadone. It is relatively convenient, with flexible dosing, ease of discontinuation, and low abuse potential. It may be best for patients with mild to moderate physical dependence and should be combined with non-pharmacological treatment services. Like methadone, buprenorphine can be used both to treat opioid withdrawal (see Figure 4.9) and as maintenance treatment. Maintenance treatment generally lasts at least 6 months and may continue for 2 years or more.

Buprenorphine/Naloxone Treatment Stages

Stage	Typical Dosage	Visits	Goal
Initiation (7 days)	After achieving mild withdrawal state: Day 1: 8 mg B/2 mg N Day 2: add'l 4 mg/1mg up to 16 mg/4 mg Days 3-7: increase in units of 4 mg/1 mg until withdrawal symptoms cease; maximum 32 mg/8 mg	At least 2 hours observation with initial dose, then 1-2 visits in first week	Achieve lowest dose that eliminates withdrawal symptoms and illicit opioid use
Stabilization (up to 2 months)	General range from 8 mg/2 mg up to 24 mg/6 mg	1/week	Eliminate withdrawal symptoms, side effects, and illicit drug use
Maintenance (based on patient needs)	Dose as determined during stabilization	Biweekly or monthly	Address lifestyle changes and social and psychological needs; if desired, plan for medically supervised withdrawal

B: buprenorphine. N: naloxone.

TABLE 4.3. Buprenorphine is commonly combined with naloxone (sublingually) in order to reduce its diversion and intravenous abuse. That is, naloxone is a mu opioid receptor antagonist that can block the effects of mu opioid agonists/partial agonists, including buprenorphine. However, because naloxone has poor sublingual bioavailability, it does not interfere with buprenorphine's effects when used properly. Naloxone does have good parenteral bioavailability; thus, if one tries to crush the tablet and administer it intravenously, naloxone will prevent any rewarding effects from buprenorphine. The dosing and treatment schedule for buprenorphine/naloxone is shown here.

DEA DATA 2000 Waiver to Prescribe Buprenorphine

DEA DATA 2000 Waiver Requirement

- Valid and current state medical license and DEA registration number
- 1 or more of the following:
    - Subspecialty board certification in addiction psychiatry from the American Board of Medical Specialties
    - Addiction certification from the American Society of Addiction Medicine
    - Subspecialty board certification in addiction medicine from the American Osteopathic Association
    - Completion of at least 8 hours of training regarding the treatment and management of opioid-addicted patients (must be sponsored by an organization authorized in the DATA 2000 legislation or another organization deemed appropriate by the Secretary of the Department of Health and Human Services)
    - Prior participation as an investigator in clinical trials leading to the approval of a Schedule III, IV, or V narcotic drug for maintenance or detoxification treatment

FIGURE 4.7. In the United States, buprenorphine can be distributed through clinicians' offices; however, practitioners who wish to prescribe it must obtain a DEA DATA 2000 waiver. The requirements for obtaining the waiver are shown in Figure 4.7. Once the waiver is obtained, practitioners can treat up to 100 patients with opioid dependence.

Naltrexone

Naltrexone
Revia, Vivitrol

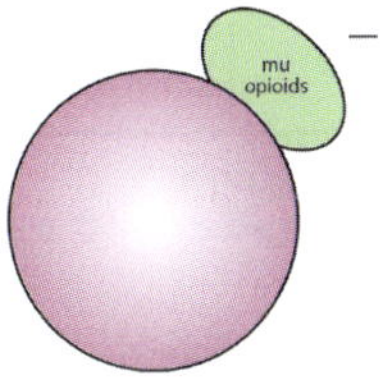

Dosage Range:
Oral: 50 mg/day or 100 mg on Mon and Wed and 150 mg on Fri
Injection: 380 mg every 4 weeks

Approved For:
Prevention of relapse to opioid dependence

Pearls:
Patients must be completely withdrawn and abstinent from opioids for 5 days (short-acting opioids) to 7 days (long-acting opioids) before starting naltrexone; common side effects include dysphoria, anxiety, gastrointestinal distress, and site reactions (injection); potential serious reactions include eosinophilic pneumonia and hepatocellular injury (at excessive doses) and serious site reactions (injection); pregnancy risk category C; contraindicated in patients with acute hepatitis or liver failure

Do not use if the patient is taking opioid analgesics, is currently dependent on opioids or is in acute opioid withdrawal, has failed the naloxone challenge, or has a positive urine screen for opioids

FIGURE 4.8. Naltrexone is a mu opioid antagonist that tightly binds to opioid receptors, blocking opioid agonists from binding there (and thus blocking their pleasurable effects) without producing a psychoactive or pleasurable effect itself. Naltrexone therefore has no abuse potential.

Because naltrexone prevents opioid agonists from binding to opioid receptors, it can precipitate an immediate withdrawal syndrome and therefore should not be given to patients who are actively dependent on opioids. Instead, before starting naltrexone, patients must be completely withdrawn and abstinent for 5 days (short-acting opioids) to 7 days (long-acting opioids).

The use of naltrexone requires a 0.8 mg IM test dose to ensure that the patient is no longer dependent on opioids before starting treatment. After discontinuing naltrexone, there is an increased sensitivity to opioid effects; thus, there is a risk that overdose will lead to respiratory depression.

Treating Opioid Withdrawal

 Methadone
Dolophine

Dosage Range:
Inpatient: usually 40–60 mg/day
Outpatient: usually higher than in inpatient treatment

Symptom Relief:
Physiological and psychological

Pearls:
In inpatient settings, detoxification can usually be achieved in 7 days for short-acting opioids; once stabilization dose is achieved, methadone can be tapered; slow tapers are associated with better outcomes; many patients tolerate reduction to 20–30 mg/day without distress

 Buprenorphine
Subutex

Dosage Range:
Inpatient: 8 mg/day
Outpatient: 8–32 mg/day

Symptom Relief:
Physiological and psychological

Pearls:
May be better accepted and more effective than clonidine; once stabilization dose is achieved, buprenorphine can be tapered in 2 mg increments over several days (longer in outpatient settings); minimal withdrawal symptoms are seen during taper; buprenorphine/naloxone combination is preferred in outpatient settings

 Clonidine
Catapres

Dosage Range:
0.1 mg 3 times daily (can be higher in inpatient setting)

Symptom Relief:
Noradrenergic (vomiting, diarrhea, cramps, and sweating)

Pearls:
Centrally acting alpha 2 adrenergic antihypertensive agent; used to suppress withdrawal symptoms when an opioid is stopped abruptly; does not reduce symptoms such as insomnia, distress, and drug cravings; detoxification can usually be achieved in 4–6 days for short-acting opioids; does not produce opioid-like tolerance or dependence; can cause hypotension; next dose should be withheld if blood pressure falls below 90/60 mm Hg; outpatients should not be given more than a 3-day supply; contraindicated in patients with cardiac disorders, renal or metabolic disease, or moderate to severe hypotension

Clonidine-Naltrexone

Pearls:
Withdrawal symptoms are precipitated by naltrexone and suppressed by clonidine; requires monitoring of the patient for 8 hours on the first day (due to potential severity of naltrexone-induced withdrawal and potential blood pressure effects of clonidine)

Treating Opioid Withdrawal (cont'd)

FIGURE 4.9. Withdrawal from opioids can include symptoms of irritability, anxiety, chills, nausea, diarrhea, sweating, sneezing, bone and muscle weakness, and insomnia. These symptoms are not life-threatening but can be severe and extremely distressing.

Medically supervised withdrawal can occur in a residential drug-free program, an inpatient detoxification unit, or an outpatient detoxification program. There are 4 main pharmacological methods for managing opioid withdrawal: methadone substitution, clonidine, buprenorphine, and clonidine/naltrexone. In addition, patients who are being treated with naltrexone for opioid dependence may receive repeated doses of naloxone with clonidine in order to shorten withdrawal during the transition between the termination of the opioid and the initiation of naltrexone.

Other medications may also be used for symptom management during opioid withdrawal. These include benzodiazepines, non-benzodiazepine sedative hypnotics, antihistamines, and sedating antidepressants for insomnia, benzodiazepines for anxiety, antiemetics for nausea and vomiting, nonsteroidal anti-inflammatory drugs (NSAIDs) for muscle cramps, and antispasmodics for gastrointestinal cramping. There is some controversy over the use of benzodiazepines during opioid withdrawal because of their abuse potential. If they are used, it should be for a short period of time (1–2 weeks).

Stahl's Illustrated | Chapter 5

Nicotine

Cigarette smoking is one of the leading causes of preventable death in the world. It is estimated that about 20% of the general population in the United States smoke. Rates are even higher in those with medical or psychiatric illnesses; 30% of individuals who regularly see a physician smoke, and 40–50% of those who see a mental health professional smoke. Yet only about 10% of smokers report being offered treatment proactively by clinicians.

This chapter reviews the neurobiological effects of nicotine as well as management strategies for patients addicted to nicotine, from screening and diagnosis to treatment selection and monitoring.

Actions of Nicotine in the VTA

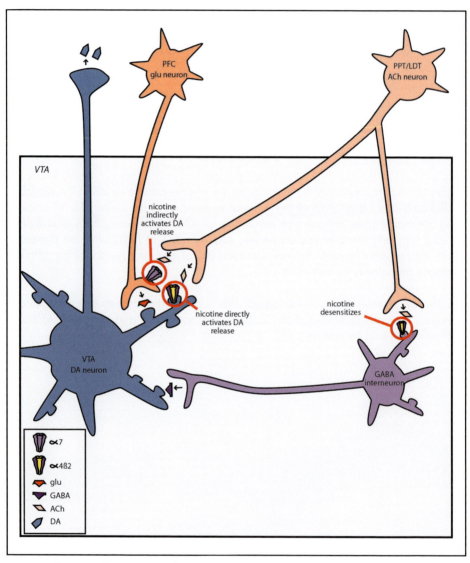

VTA: ventral tegmental area. PFC: prefrontal cortex. glu: glutamate. PPT/LDT: pedunculopontine and laterodorsal tegmental nucleus. ACh: acetylcholine. DA: dopamine. GABA: gamma aminobutyric acid.

Actions of Nicotine in the VTA (cont'd)

FIGURE 5.1. Nicotine acts directly on nicotinic cholinergic receptors in the VTA. There are 2 major subtypes of nicotinic receptors that are known to be present in the brain: the alpha 4 beta 2 subtype and the alpha 7 subtype.

Nicotine directly causes dopamine release in the nucleus accumbens by binding to alpha 4 beta 2 nicotinic postsynaptic receptors on dopamine neurons in the VTA. In addition, nicotine binds to alpha 7 nicotinic presynaptic receptors on glutamate neurons in the VTA, which in turn leads to dopamine release in the nucleus accumbens. Nicotine also seems to desensitize alpha 4 beta 2 postsynaptic receptors on GABA interneurons in the VTA; the reduction of GABA neurotransmission disinhibits mesolimbic dopamine neurons and is thus a third mechanism for enhancing dopamine release in the nucleus accumbens.

Reinforcement and Alpha 4 Beta 2 Nicotinic Receptors

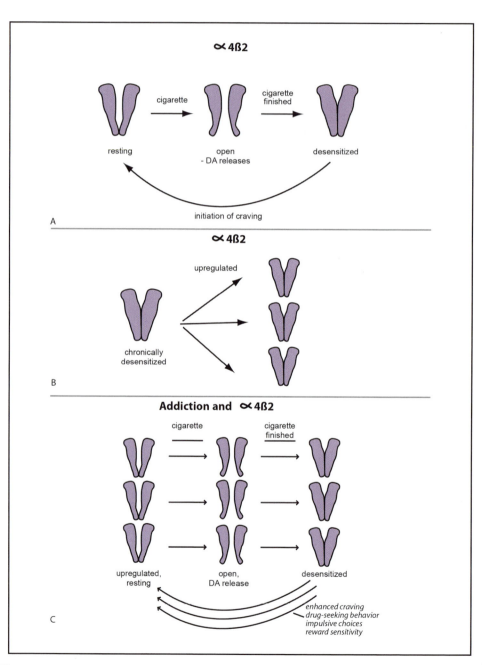

Reinforcement and Alpha 4 Beta 2 Nicotinic Receptors (cont'd)

FIGURE 5.2. The alpha 4 beta 2 nicotinic receptors on dopamine neurons in the VTA are thought to be the primary targets of nicotine's reinforcing properties. These receptors adapt to the chronic intermittent pulsatile delivery of nicotine in a way that leads to addiction.

(A) In the resting state, alpha 4 beta 2 nicotinic receptors are closed (left). Nicotine administration, as by smoking a cigarette, causes the receptor to open, which in turn leads to dopamine release (middle). Long-term stimulation of these receptors leads to their desensitization, such that they temporarily cannot react to nicotine (or to acetylcholine); this occurs in approximately the same amount of time it takes to finish a single cigarette (right).

(B) With chronic desensitization, alpha 4 beta 2 nicotinic receptors upregulate to compensate.

(C) If one continues smoking, however, the repeated administration of nicotine continues to lead to desensitization of all of these alpha 4 beta 2 receptors, and thus, the upregulation does no good. In fact, the upregulation can lead to amplified craving as the extra receptors resensitize to their resting state.

Nicotine's Consequences:
A Function of the Delivery System

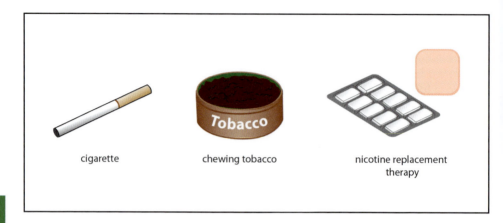

FIGURE 5.3. The negative health consequences of nicotine use vary based on the method of intake. As shown in Figure 2.3, the mode of delivery has an impact on the addictive potential, with the inhalation of nicotine through cigarettes as the most addictive method. Unfortunately, the negative health effects of nicotine consumption are also the greatest for cigarettes: although chewing tobacco and snuff deliver higher nicotine levels to the blood than cigarettes, they only modestly raise the risk for cardiovascular disease or cancer in comparison to cigarettes, which cause a substantial increase in lung cancer, heart disease, and chronic obstructive pulmonary disease. Nicotine replacement therapy has minimal cardiovascular effects and no apparent detrimental effect on lung function or cancer risk.

Brief Intervention for Smoking Cessation

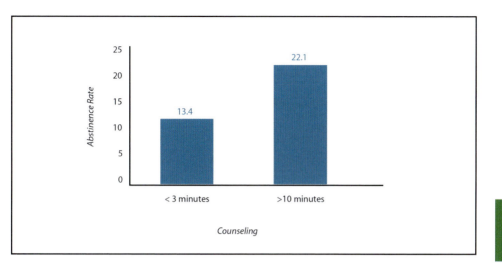

FIGURE 5.4. Although as many as 70% of smokers express a desire to quit, only 2.5% are successful each year. Individuals who have assistance from a health care professional are twice as likely to quit smoking as those without assistance. Even just asking patients about their willingness to quit smoking may increase the likelihood of successful cessation, and data show that brief counseling (3 minutes or less) significantly increases the odds of prolonged abstinence. A longer counseling session (10 minutes or more) doubles the odds compared to minimal counseling.

All patients should be asked about their tobacco use, and all patients who use tobacco should be advised to quit. This involves assessing each patient's readiness to quit, and, if they are ready to make a quit attempt, assisting them with counseling and pharmacotherapy as well as arranging follow-up support. These steps are called the 5 As (ask, advise, assess, assist, arrange).

For patients who are not ready to attempt smoking cessation, remind them that you are available to help them when they are ready, and be sure to ask at subsequent visits.

Management Strategy for Smoking Cessation

1
- Congratulate
- Set quit date (in 2–6 weeks)
- Discuss medication options
- Identify strategies to enhance success
- Refer to 1-800-QUIT NOW
- Set appointment for 1–2 weeks before quit date

2
Pre-quit appointment:
- Reinforce the decision to quit and the need for abstinence
- Discuss interaction with nicotine dependence counselor, if applicable
- Prescribe medication, discussing side effects and the importance of adherence
- Set follow-up appointment for 1–2 weeks after quit date (can be by phone)

3
Follow-up appointment:
- Listen carefully to challenges and possible lapses
- Reinforce the decision to quit and the need for abstinence
- Encourage adherence
- Tailor duration of treatment to cravings/side effects

FIGURE 5.5. For patients who are ready to attempt to quit, a quit date should be set for some time in the next few weeks. In addition to discussing pharmacological options, one should work with the patient to identify strategies that may enhance success, such as how to avoid certain triggers. If the patient has had previous quit attempts, discuss what was or was not previously helpful. Another appointment should be scheduled for 1–2 weeks before the quit date, at which point a medication should be prescribed with full explanation of its side effects and guidelines for use as well as the importance of adherence.

Follow-up appointments should be scheduled for a couple of weeks after the quit date and then monthly for a few months (phone consult is fine). The duration of treatment can be determined based on the patient's progress over this time period. Nicotine dependence is very difficult to overcome, and most patients will attempt to quit multiple times before achieving success.

Pharmacological Treatment for Smoking Cessation

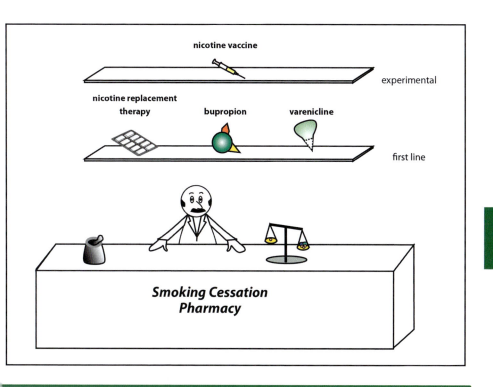

FIGURE 5.6. The Surgeon General recommends that every patient attempting to quit smoking should receive a pharmacological treatment. Options include various formulations of nicotine replacement therapy, bupropion, and varenicline. These treatments can also be combined with one another. Though not extensively studied, there is some evidence of increased efficacy of varenicline plus bupropion compared with either treatment alone. There are also positive data suggesting the benefits of combining nicotine replacement therapy with another agent, including a study in which the combination of 2 different nicotine replacement formulations (i.e., the patch and the lozenge) resulted in higher abstinence rates (relative to placebo) than the 4 other monotherapies studied. In another study, the combination of the nicotine patch, the nicotine inhaler, and bupropion resulted in higher abstinence rates than treatment with the patch alone.

The most promising investigational agent for smoking cessation is currently a nicotine vaccine, which is being studied in Phase III trials.

Psychosocial Treatment for Nicotine Dependence

		CBT	MET	Behavioral therapy	IPT	Family therapy	Self-help/ 12-step
Substance of Abuse	Alcohol	X	X	X		X	X
	Opioid	X		X		X	X
	Nicotine	X	X	X			
	Stimulant	X		X			X
	THC		X	X			

CBT: cognitive behavioral therapy. MET: motivational enhancement therapy. Behavioral therapy: contingency management, community reinforcement, cue exposure and relaxation, aversion therapy. IPT: interpersonal therapy. THC: delta-9-tetrahydrocannabinol.

Psychosocial Treatment for Nicotine Dependence (cont'd)

TABLE 5.1. Psychosocial strategies can be used as adjuncts to support efforts to quit and include motivational enhancement therapy, behavioral therapies, and cognitive behavioral therapy. These methods are also used by individuals with other substance use disorders and are described in more detail in Chapter 9. Social support is also an extremely important part of treatment for smoking cessation.

Additional resources for patients include telephone quit lines and local cessation centers. 1-800-QUIT-NOW is a free national call line established by the United States Department of Health and Human Services. Patients who call this number are routed to a trained cessation counselor who takes a complete history and helps develop a quitting strategy. Local cessation centers and programs offer tobacco cessation counseling and education and are offered at many large hospitals as well as through chapters of the American Cancer Society, the American Heart Association, and the American Lung Association. The cost and duration of the programs offered can vary.

Although patients may be referred to quit lines or local cessation centers, prescription pharmacotherapy may not be available through these means; thus, determination of the best pharmacological approach for the patient may affect whether or not these resources can be used as the sole source of treatment.

Nicotine Replacement Therapy (NRT)

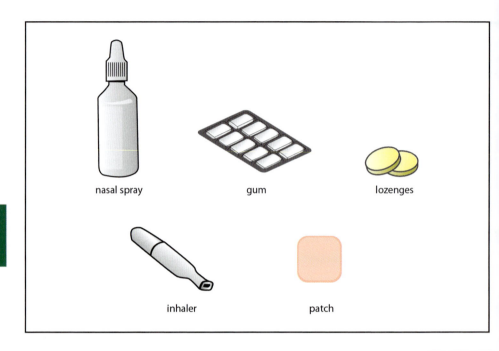

FIGURE 5.7. There are 5 major formulations available for nicotine replacement therapies: gum, patch, nasal spray, inhaler, and lozenge. Individuals must stop smoking before initiating any nicotine replacement therapy. Nicotine replacement therapy should be used cautiously in individuals with cardiovascular disease and avoided in patients with unstable coronary artery disease.

The pregnancy category for all nicotine replacement therapies is D. For pregnant women who smoke heavily and are motivated to quit but have been unsuccessful using nonpharmacological methods, the risks of continuing smoking may outweigh the risks of using nicotine replacement therapy; however, other treatment options are available and should be considered first.

Nicotine Gum

Nicotine gum
Nicorette

Dosage Range:
9–12 pieces per day (2 mg or 4 mg per piece)

Duration of Treatment:
Typically 6 weeks, then taper, though longer treatment may be beneficial

Advantages:
Flexible dosing

Disadvantages:
Requires frequent dosing; no food/drink 15 minutes before use; use caution in patients with dental problems or temporomandibular joint pain syndrome

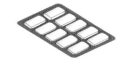

FIGURE 5.8. Nicotine gum is available over the counter in strengths of 2 mg (for those who smoke less than 25 cigarettes per day) or 4 mg (for those who smoke 25 or more cigarettes per day). Nicotine absorption peaks after approximately 30 minutes with the gum, which should be chewed until a tingling sensation occurs, after which it should be "parked" between the cheek and the gum. Food or drink (acidic beverages in particular) should not be consumed for 15 minutes prior to use. A piece of gum is typically chewed every 1–2 waking hours during the first 6 weeks, after which the frequency may be tapered. No more than 30 pieces of the 2-mg dose or 20 pieces of the 4-mg dose should be chewed in a single day. Adverse effects include jaw pain, sore throat, excess saliva, oral blisters, nausea, and indigestion. In addition, the saliva should not be swallowed, as it can cause heartburn or gastrointestinal irritation. Approximately 10% of individuals using the gum develop dependence.

Nicotine Patch

Nicotine patch
Nicoderm 24H, Nicotrol 16H

Dosage Range:
1 patch per day (7, 15 ,or 21 mg per 24-hour patch; 5, 10, or 15 mg per 16-hour patch)

Duration of Treatment:
Typically 6 weeks, then taper, though longer treatment may be beneficial

Advantages:
Once-daily dosing; overnight use may control morning cravings

Disadvantages:
Dosing not flexible; can cause sleep problems if worn at night

FIGURE 5.9. The nicotine transdermal patch is available in multiple formulations, 2 of which can be obtained over the counter. The patch is administered once daily and is available in a 16-hour or 24-hour duration; the site where the patch is placed should be rotated. The 16-hour patch causes less sleep disturbance, while the 24-hour patch provides greater control of early morning cravings. Daily plasma concentrations of nicotine peak after 4–8 hours, and steady state concentration is reached after 2–3 days of use. Available doses are 7 mg, 14 mg, and 21 mg (24-hour release) and 5 mg, 10 mg, and 15 mg (16-hour release). The lower doses may be used in a stepdown approach or in patients who are light smokers; heavy smokers should use the 21-mg dose. The most common adverse effects are site reactions; medium potency steroid cream can be prescribed to alleviate skin irritation. The risk of dependence with the transdermal patch is lower than that with nicotine gum. The nicotine patch is the least expensive of the available nicotine replacement therapies, although no nicotine replacement therapy is as expensive as purchasing cigarettes.

Nicotine Nasal Spray

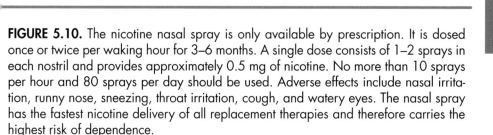

Nicotine nasal spray
Nicotrol NS

Dosage Range:
1–2 times per waking hour (0.5 mg per dose)

Duration of Treatment:
Typically 3–6 months, then taper, though longer treatment may be beneficial

Advantages:
Flexible dosing

Disadvantages:
Requires frequent dosing; highest risk of dependence of all NRTs

FIGURE 5.10. The nicotine nasal spray is only available by prescription. It is dosed once or twice per waking hour for 3–6 months. A single dose consists of 1–2 sprays in each nostril and provides approximately 0.5 mg of nicotine. No more than 10 sprays per hour and 80 sprays per day should be used. Adverse effects include nasal irritation, runny nose, sneezing, throat irritation, cough, and watery eyes. The nasal spray has the fastest nicotine delivery of all replacement therapies and therefore carries the highest risk of dependence.

Nicotine Inhaler

Nicotine Inhaler
Nicotrol Inhaler

Dosage Range:
6–16 cartridges per day (4 mg per dose)

Duration of Treatment:
Typically 3 months, then taper, though longer treatment may be beneficial

Advantages:
Flexible dosing; mimics hand-to-mouth gesture of smoking

Disadvantages:
Requires frequent dosing

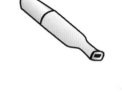

FIGURE 5.11. Like the nicotine nasal spray, the inhaler is only available by prescription. The inhaler consists of a cartridge attached to a mouthpiece, with each cartridge delivering a 4-mg dose of nicotine. Patients typically use 6–16 cartridges per day for 3 months, after which the dose can be tapered over another 6 months. Although administered with an inhaler, the nicotine is actually absorbed in the mouth as opposed to in the lungs; thus, delivery to the brain is slower than with the nasal spray, creating a lower risk of dependence. Adverse effects include mouth irritation, cough, headache, nausea, and bronchospasm. Benefits of the nicotine inhaler include the fact that it mimics the hand-to-mouth motion of smoking and that it has few adverse effects, such as mild throat irritation and cough.

Nicotine Oral Lozenge

Nicotine lozenge
Commit

Dosage Range:
9 lozenges per day (2 or 4 mg per dose)

Duration of Treatment:
Typically 6 weeks, then taper, though longer treatment may be beneficial

Advantages:
Flexible dosing

Disadvantages:
Requires frequent dosing; no food/drinks 15 minutes before use

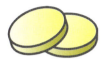

FIGURE 5.12. The nicotine lozenge is available in 2-mg and 4-mg doses and is typically dosed as 9 lozenges per day. Individuals who generally smoke within 30 minutes of waking should use the 4-mg dose. The lozenge should be placed in the mouth and allowed to dissolve, which takes approximately 20–30 minutes. In comparison with the nicotine gum, the lozenge delivers approximately 25% more nicotine per dose. As with the gum, no food or drink should be consumed within 15 minutes of use. Adverse effects include mouth soreness, dyspepsia, nausea, and headache.

Bupropion

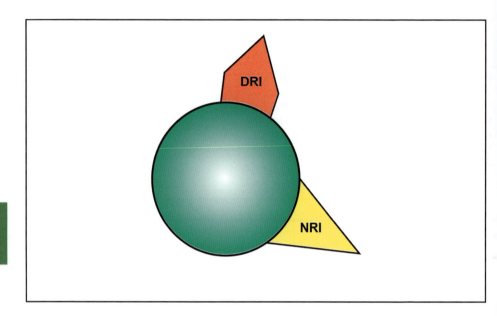

FIGURE 5.13. Bupropion is a norepinephrine and dopamine reuptake inhibitor that can alleviate cravings during smoking cessation. When an individual smokes chronically, the regular nicotine intake leads to dopamine release in the nucleus accumbens; thus, during smoking cessation, there is a deficit of dopamine, which contributes to cravings and what some call a "nicotine fit." By blocking dopamine reuptake directly in the nucleus accumbens, bupropion is able to increase the availability of that neurotransmitter. Although not as powerful as nicotine, it does take the edge off and can make abstinence more tolerable.

Bupropion (Zyban):
Tips and Pearls

Dosing and Use

Formulation:
Sustained release tablet: 100 mg, 150 mg, 200 mg; other formulations are also available

Dosing for Smoking Cessation (sustained release):
Initial 150 mg/day, after 3 days increase to 300 mg/day in 2 doses

Approved For:
Nicotine addiction (SR); major depressive disorder; seasonal affective disorder (XL)

Side Effects and Safety

Weight Gain

unusual — not unusual — common — problematic

Sedation

unusual — not unusual — common — problematic

 Rare: suicidal ideation and behavior, hypomania, seizures

 Do not use if patient has a history of seizures, is anorexic or bulimic, is abruptly discontinuing alcohol or sedatives, has had a head injury, has a nervous system tumor, is taking an MAOI or thioridazine, or is taking any other formulation of bupropion

Pearls

 Should be initiated 2 weeks before smoking discontinuation; can be used in conjunction with nicotine replacement therapy; do not break or chew SR or XL tablets, as this will alter their controlled release properties; use cautiously with other drugs that increase seizure risk; if insomnia occurs, do not give the second dose past mid-afternoon

Special Populations

 Safety and efficacy have not been established; may be used for smoking cessation in adolescents

 Pregnancy risk category C (some animal studies show adverse effects; no controlled studies in humans)

 Limited available data on patients with cardiac impairment; evidence of rise in supine blood pressure

 Drug concentration may be increased in renal impairment; lower initial dose and perhaps give less frequently

 Lower initial dose and perhaps give less frequently

FIGURE 5.14. Dosing and safety information for bupropion.

Varenicline

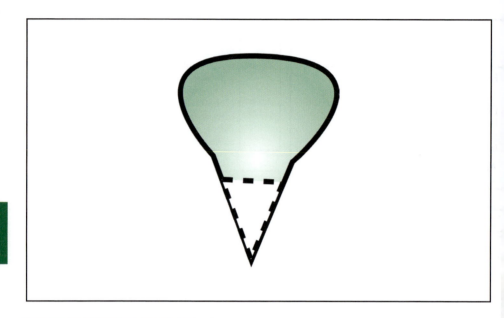

FIGURE 5.15. Varenicline is an alpha 4 beta 2 nicotinic receptor partial agonist. Like other smoking cessation options, varenicline has the potential to reduce withdrawal symptoms in the absence of smoking by providing drug-induced neurotransmission. However, unlike other smoking cessation treatments, varenicline can also prevent the "dopaminergic" reward that normally occurs in the event that a patient does smoke. This is because varenicline binds to the same receptors as nicotine so that it can compete with nicotine for the receptors and thereby reduce its effects.

Varenicline (Chantix):
Tips and Pearls

Dosing and Use

Formulation:
Tablet: 0.5 mg, 1 mg

Dosing:
Initial 0.5 mg/day; after 3 days increase to 1 mg/day in two doses; after 4 more days increase to 2 mg/day in 2 doses

Approved For:
Nicotine addiction/dependence

Side Effects and Safety

Weight Gain

unusual   not unusual   common   problematic

Sedation

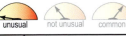

unusual   not unusual   common   problematic

 Rare: suicidal ideation and behavior, agitation, depressed mood

 No contraindications other than proven allergy to varenicline

Pearls

 Should be initiated 1 week before smoking discontinuation; should be taken following a meal and with a full glass of water; may reduce both the withdrawal effects and the reinforcing effects of nicotine; cannot be "smoked over" because it blocks the same receptors as nicotine; side effects may be increased if it is taken with nicotine replacement therapy

Special Populations

 Safety and efficacy have not been established

 Pregnancy risk category C (some animal studies show adverse effects; no controlled studies in humans)

 Limited available data on patients with cardiac impairment

 For severe renal impairment, maximum recommended dose is 0.5 mg twice per day; for patients with end-stage renal disease undergoing hemodialysis, maximum recommended dose is 0.5 mg once per day; removed by hemodialysis

 Dose adjustment not generally necessary for patients with hepatic impairment

FIGURE 5.16. Dosing and safety information for varenicline.

Stahl's Illustrated

Chapter 6

Stimulants

The misuse of stimulants is a significant public health problem. Although therapeutic stimulants such as methylphenidate and amphetamine can be—and are—abused, the evolution of controlled release technology has somewhat helped to curb this problem. The abuse of cocaine and methamphetamine, however, continues to be a rampant problem. This chapter covers the neurobiology of stimulant use and abuse, the mechanisms of action of stimulants, and management strategies for patients with stimulant use disorder. It should be noted that the majority of data exist for cocaine dependence; however, pharmacotherapy for methamphetamine dependence is expected to be similar.

Actions of Stimulants on Reward Circuits

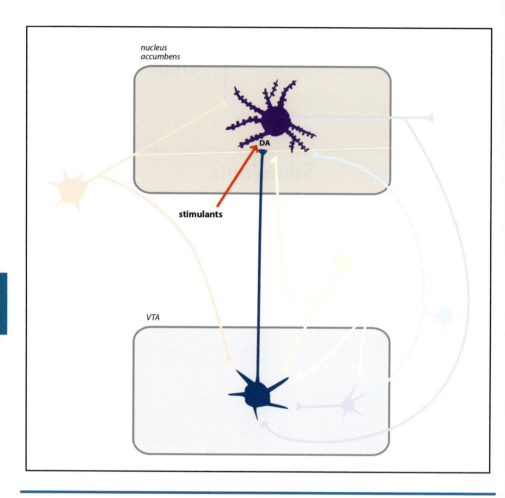

FIGURE 6.1. The potential abuse properties of stimulants stem from their ability to enhance dopamine neurotransmission in the nucleus accumbens. Therapeutic stimulants include methylphenidate and amphetamine; illicit stimulants include cocaine and methamphetamine.

Cocaine (and Methylphenidate) vs. Methamphetamine (and Amphetamine), Part 1

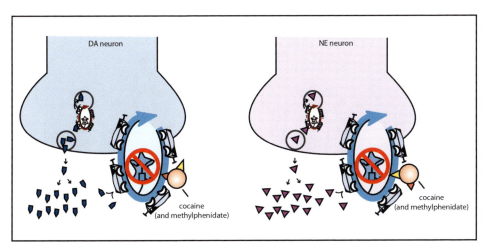

FIGURE 6.2. Stimulants such as cocaine and methamphetamine increase synaptic dopamine and norepinephrine levels by blocking their respective transporters. However, although this is the primary mechanism of action of cocaine, methamphetamine also enhances dopamine release, especially at high doses.

Cocaine (and Methylphenidate) vs. Methamphetamine (and Amphetamine), Part 2

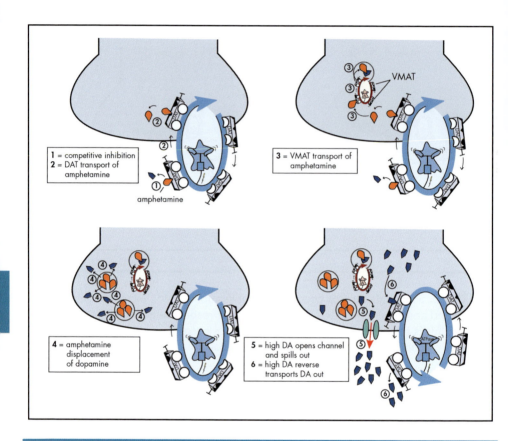

FIGURE 6.3. Unlike cocaine, methamphetamine is a competitive inhibitor of the dopamine transporter; thus, it competes with DA for a seat on the transporter (1). By hijacking the dopamine transporter, methamphetamine itself is transported into the DA terminal (2).

Methamphetamine is also a competitive inhibitor of the vesicular monoamine transporter (VMAT), located inside the DA terminal (3). It is therefore able to be packaged into vesicles (3). At high levels, methamphetamine will displace DA from the vesicles into the terminal (4). Once a critical threshold of DA has been reached, DA will be expelled from the terminal via 2 mechanisms: the opening of channels to allow for a massive dumping of DA into the synapse (5) and the reversal of the dopamine transporter (6).

What Gives a Stimulant its Abuse Potential?

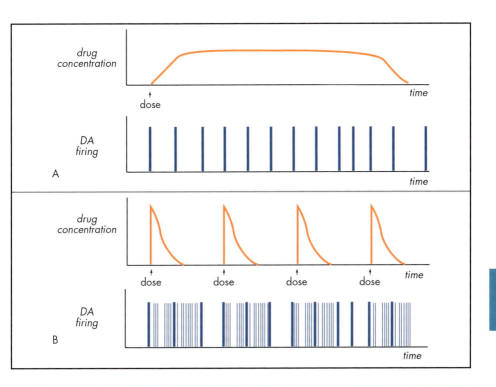

FIGURE 6.4. As shown in Figure 2.3, the reinforcing effects of drugs are largely determined by the rate at which DA increases in the brain, which in turn is dictated by the speed at which the drug enters and leaves the brain. The rate of drug uptake is subject to the route of administration, with intravenous administration and inhalation producing the fastest drug uptake, followed by snorting.

Methylphenidate and amphetamine are given orally and have a longer onset and duration of action compared to cocaine and methamphetamine (A). Although they can be abused if injected or snorted rather than taken orally, the controlled release formulations that are now commonly prescribed make this more difficult.

Cocaine and methamphetamine, by contrast, are generally administered intravenously, by smoking, or by snorting. In fact, cocaine is not even active orally. Correspondingly, cocaine and methamphetamine cause a rapid increase in DA, followed by a relatively rapid decline (B).

Progression of Stimulant Abuse

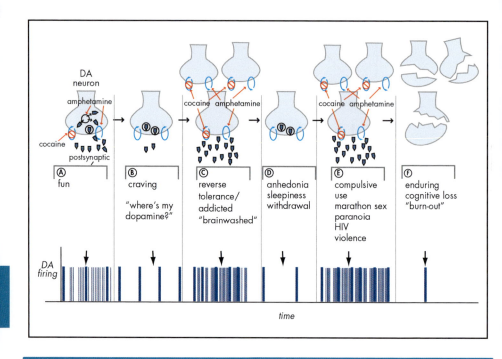

FIGURE 6.5. Initial doses of stimulants such as methamphetamine and cocaine cause pleasurable phasic dopamine firing (A). With chronic use, reward conditioning causes craving between stimulant doses and residual tonic dopamine firing with a lack of pleasurable phasic dopamine firing (B). In this addicted state, higher and higher doses of stimulants are needed in order to achieve the pleasurable highs of phasic dopamine firing (C). Unfortunately, the higher the high, the lower the low, and between stimulant doses, the individual experiences not only the absence of a high, but also withdrawal symptoms such as sleepiness and anhedonia (D). The effort to combat withdrawal can lead to compulsive use and impulsive, dangerous behavior in order to secure the stimulant (E). Finally, there may be enduring if not irreversible changes in dopamine neurons, including long-lasting depletions of dopamine levels and axonal degeneration, a state that clinically and pathologically is appropriately called "burn-out" (F).

Stimulant Effects

No treatment or beta blocker or DA antagonist

No treatment or benzodiazepine

No treatment or antipsychotic

FIGURE 6.6. Cocaine and methamphetamine can cause euphoria and pleasure, reduce fatigue, and create a sense of mental acuity. Undesirable effects can also be produced, however, and include tremor, emotional lability, restlessness, irritability, paranoia, panic, and repetitive stereotyped behavior. At higher doses, these stimulants can induce intense anxiety, paranoia, and hallucinations along with hypertension, tachycardia, ventricular irritability, hyperthermia, and respiratory depression. In overdose, cocaine can cause acute heart failure, stroke, and seizures.

The treatment of stimulant intoxication is generally supportive and addresses autonomic hyperactivity as well as paranoia and hallucinations, if necessary. However, many patients will recovery within hours without treatment. Treatments that have been used or investigated include beta blockers and dopamine antagonists for cardiovascular effects, benzodiazepines for extreme agitation, and antipsychotics for paranoia and hallucinations. Caution should be exercised if these agents are used.

Cocaethylene

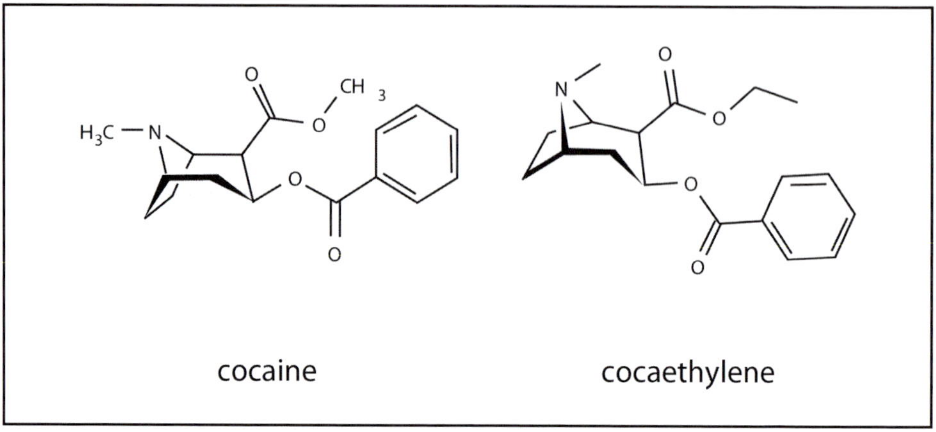

cocaine   cocaethylene

FIGURE 6.7. A unique drug interaction can occur between cocaine and ethanol in which the 2 substances form the metabolite cocaethylene, which has cocaine-like effects but is more toxic and has a longer half-life than cocaine. Animal studies have documented the deleterious hemodynamic and cardiovascular effects of cocaethylene, and human data also suggest an increased risk of complications.

Pharmacological Treatment for Stimulant Use Disorder

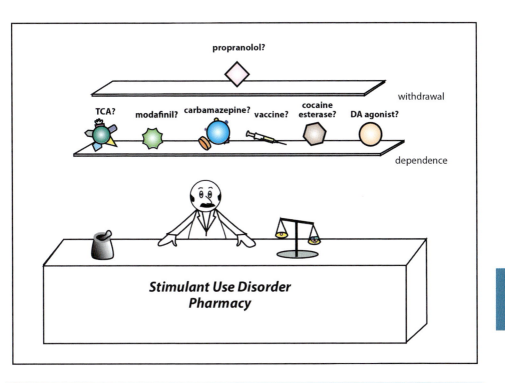

FIGURE 6.8. There is little evidence for the pharmacological treatment of stimulant dependence or withdrawal. Most studies have specifically investigated treatment options for cocaine dependence. Dopamine agonists (amantadine in particular) are the best studied for this use; however, data are generally mixed, with some studies showing trends in favor of dopamine agonists and others favoring placebo. Overall, the existing evidence does not support their use.

Meta-analysis of existing trials evaluating anticonvulsants as treatments for cocaine dependence did not show significant efficacy for any of the agents included. At best, carbamazepine showed a trend toward higher retention rates (i.e., continuation of anticonvulsant treatment) than placebo. Antidepressants have been studied in the treatment of cocaine dependence, but the current data do not support their use (some studies show trends in favor of tricyclic antidepressants). There is also preliminary study of modafinil, investigation of a potential cocaine vaccine, and investigation of a cocaine-metabolizing enzyme (cocaine esterase).

Psychosocial Treatment for Stimulant Use Disorder

		CBT	MET	Behavioral therapy	IPT	Family therapy	Self-help/ 12-step
Substance of Abuse	Alcohol	X	X	X		X	X
	Opioid	X		X		X	X
	Nicotine	X	X	X			
	Stimulant	X		X			X
	THC		X	X			

CBT: cognitive behavioral therapy. MET: motivational enhancement therapy. Behavioral therapy: contingency management, community reinforcement, cue exposure and relaxation, aversion therapy. IPT: interpersonal therapy. THC: delta-9-tetrahydrocannabinol.

TABLE 6.1. Psychosocial treatments are an extremely important component of substance use disorder management. Many of the same general strategies are used to treat addiction to/dependence on different substances of abuse. The specific strategies that are commonly used in the treatment of stimulant use disorder are highlighted here. CBT is particularly effective for more severe cases and those with comorbid disorders. Twelve-step facilitation and individual drug counseling can also be effective. These strategies are explained in more detail in Chapter 9.

Stimulant Withdrawal

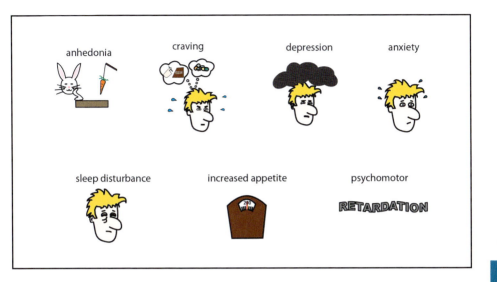

FIGURE 6.9. Abstinence from cocaine or methamphetamine use does not always cause specific withdrawal symptoms. When symptoms do occur, they typically begin within a few hours to several days of acute cessation, and may include anhedonia, cocaine cravings, depression, anxiety, sleep disturbance, increased appetite, and psychomotor retardation. Symptoms typically decline over several weeks and do not generally require inpatient treatment.

Currently, there are no recommended pharmacological treatments for patients experiencing stimulant-related withdrawal symptoms. Preliminary data suggest that propranolol may have efficacy for patients with severe withdrawal symptoms.

Experimental Treatments for Cocaine Dependence

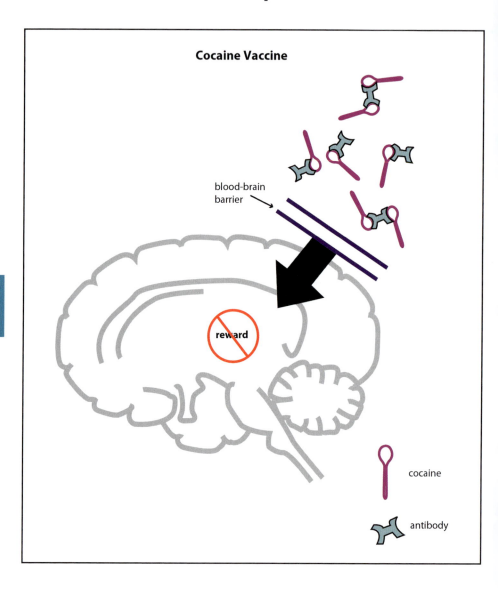

Experimental Treatments for Cocaine Dependence (cont'd)

FIGURE 6.10. Although there are no established effective treatments for cocaine dependence, there are 2 promising areas of research: cocaine esterase and a cocaine vaccine.

Cocaine esterase is an enzyme that metabolizes cocaine. A bacterial cocaine esterase (CocE) has established efficacy for treating the acute toxic effects of cocaine overdose; however, its half-life is too short for it to be used as a maintenance treatment for cocaine dependence. Thus, a mutant CocE (PEG-CCRQ CocE) with a longer half-life has been developed and has tested positively in animal models.

A cocaine vaccine is also in development. Formulation of a vaccine for cocaine requires coupling it to a carrier molecule, as the cocaine molecule is too small to elicit an immune response. The antibodies produced in response to the vaccine do not cross into the brain; thus, antibody-bound cocaine remains in the periphery and the reinforcing effects of cocaine administration may be attenuated. Studies of the cocaine vaccine dAd5GNE have shown positive results in animal models.

Stahl's Illustrated | Chapter 7

Marijuana

Marijuana is the most widely used substance of abuse in the world. It has less dependence potential than other major substances of abuse; however, its abuse can be associated with social, cognitive, and other problems, including an increased risk of other substance use. Unfortunately, research into the treatment of marijuana dependence has been limited. This chapter covers what is known about the neurobiology and treatment of marijuana use disorder.

Actions of Marijuana and THC on Reward Circuits

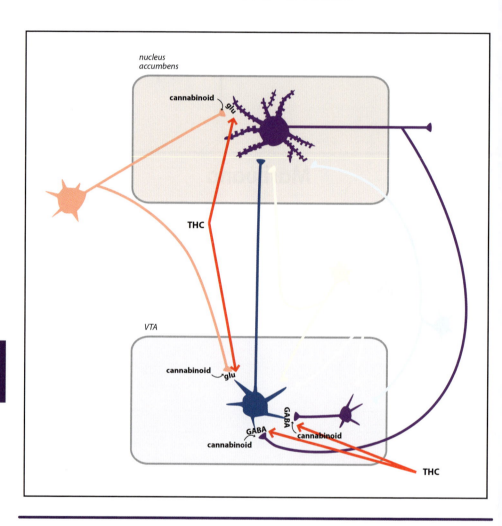

FIGURE 7.1. The active ingredients in marijuana are cannabinoids, with delta-9-tetrahydrocannabinol (THC) primarily responsible for marijuana's effects. THC interacts with cannabinoid 1 receptors in the VTA and the nucleus accumbens to trigger dopamine release from mesolimbic neurons.

Cannabinoids are Retrograde Neurotransmitters

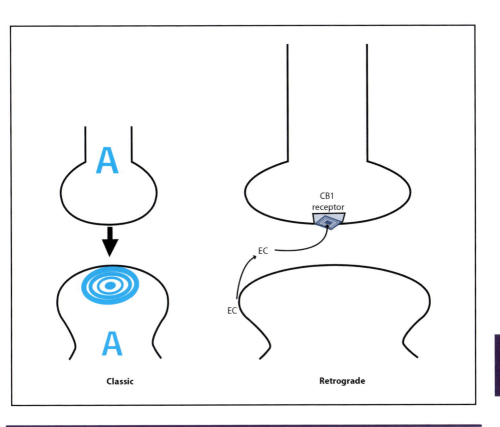

FIGURE 7.2. Endocannabinoids (EC, or endogenous marijuana) are retrograde neurotransmitters. That is, instead of exhibiting classic neurotransmission from pre- to postsynaptic neurons (left), endocannabinoids are synthesized in the postsynaptic neuron, released, and diffuse to presynaptic cannabinoid receptors such as the CB1 receptor, thus allowing postsynaptic neurons to communicate back to presynaptic neurons (right).

Effects of Marijuana

Intoxication	High Dose	Long-Term Heavy Use
Well-being	Panic	Amotivation
Relaxation	Toxic delirium	Poor attention span
Friendliness	Psychosis (rare)	Poor judgment
Special insight		Distractibilty
Temporally unaware		Poor communication
Slow thought processes		Introversion
Impaired memory		Poor interpersonal skills
		Loss of insight
		Depersonalization

FIGURE 7.3. Marijuana can have both stimulant and sedative properties. In usual intoxicating doses, it produces a sense of well-being, relaxation, friendliness, and a feeling of achieving special insights. It also induces a loss of temporal awareness (e.g., confusing the past with the present), a slowing of thought processes, and impairment of short-term memory. At high doses, marijuana can induce panic, toxic delirium, and rarely psychosis.

One complication of long-term, heavy, frequent use is the "amotivational syndrome," which is characterized by the emergence of decreased drive and ambition. Heavy marijuana use is also associated with other socially and occupationally impairing symptoms, including a shortened attention span, poor judgment, easy distractibility, impaired communication skills, introversion, and diminished effectiveness in interpersonal situations. Personal habits may deteriorate, and there may be a loss of insight and even feelings of depersonalization.

Pharmacologic Treatment for Marijuana Use Disorder

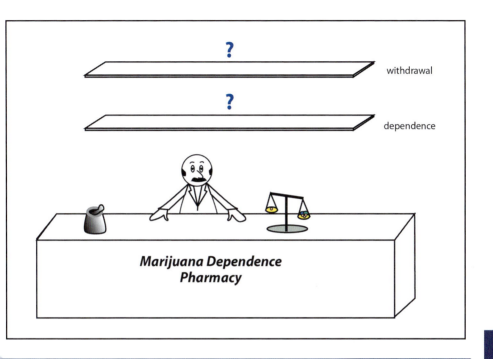

FIGURE 7.4. There is little evidence for the pharmacological treatment of marijuana dependence or withdrawal, and no pharmacotherapies are recommended.

Psychosocial Treatment for Marijuana Use Disorder

		CBT	MET	Behavioral therapy	IPT	Family therapy	Self-help/ 12-step
Substance of Abuse	Alcohol	X	X	X		X	X
	Opioid	X		X		X	X
	Nicotine	X	X	X			
	Stimulant	X		X			X
	THC		X	X			

CBT: cognitive behavioral therapy. MET: motivational enhancement therapy. Behavioral therapy: contingency management, community reinforcement, cue exposure and relaxation, aversion therapy. IPT: interpersonal therapy. THC: delta-9-tetrahydrocannabinol.

TABLE 7.1. Psychosocial treatments are an extremely important component of substance use disorder management. Many of the same general strategies are used to treat addiction to/dependence on different substances of abuse. The specific strategies that are commonly used in the treatment of marijuana use disorder are highlighted here. A motivational enhancement approach that incorporates coping skills may be most effective; using incentives can also be valuable. These strategies are explained in more detail in Chapter 9.

Marijuana Withdrawal

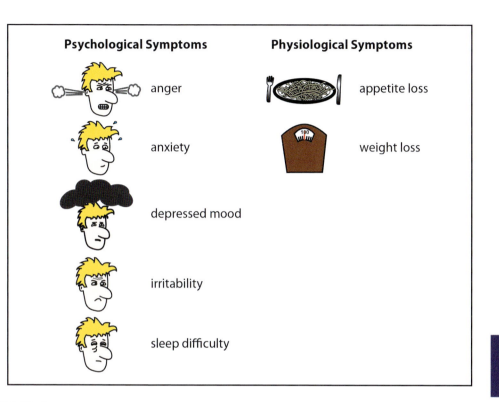

FIGURE 7.5. Although marijuana is considered by many to be a substance that can be easily stopped at any time, in actuality, it can cause dependence in heavy users and therefore withdrawal symptoms when discontinued. Psychological symptoms are most common and include anger, anxiety, depressed mood, irritability, and sleep difficulty. Physiological symptoms may also occur, such as appetite and weight loss.

There is currently no pharmacotherapy specifically recommended for either marijuana withdrawal or the maintenance of abstinence following marijuana cessation. Bupropion, divalproex, and naltrexone have all been studied in human trials of marijuana withdrawal, but all the trials have had negative results. Dronabinol, a synthetic formulation of THC, has been preliminarily studied for marijuana withdrawal, but current results are not sufficient to recommend its use. Instead, marijuana dependence and any associated withdrawal is usually treated with psychosocial therapies, as shown in Table 7.1. Withdrawal symptoms typically resolve within 1–2 weeks.

Stahl's Illustrated | Chapter 8

Other Drugs of Abuse

Many other substances are abused for their reinforcing properties. These agents, which include sedative hypnotics, hallucinogens, "club drugs," designer drugs, and even ordinary household products, may not have the addictive potential of some of the agents discussed in previous chapters; however, they are all extremely dangerous. This chapter briefly covers how these agents work as well as the effects that they can have.

SECTION ONE:
Sedative Hypnotics

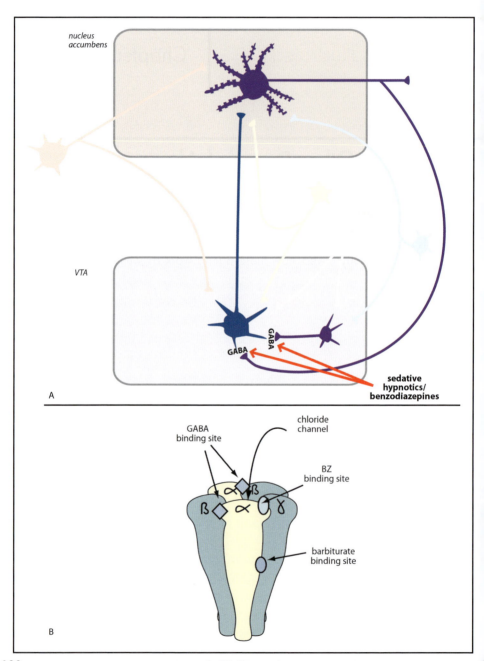

SECTION ONE:
Sedative Hypnotics (cont'd)

FIGURE 8.1. Sedative hypnotics include barbiturates and related agents such as ethchlorvynol and ethinamate, chloral hydrate and derivatives, and piperidinedione derivatives such as glutethimide and methyprylon. Experts often include alcohol, benzodiazepines, and Z drug hypnotics in this class as well. Benzodiazepines and barbiturates are positive allosteric modulators (PAMs) of GABA-A receptors (A). Benzodiazepines and barbiturates both act at GABA-A receptors, but at different binding sites (B).

Compared with benzodiazepines, barbiturates are much less safe in overdose, cause dependence more frequently, are abused more frequently, and produce much more dangerous withdrawal reactions. Apparently, the receptor site at GABA-A receptors that mediates the pharmacological actions of barbiturates is even more readily desensitized, and with even more dangerous consequences, than the benzodiazepine receptor site. The barbiturate site also seems to mediate a more intense euphoria and a more desirable sense of tranquility than the benzodiazepine receptor site. Since benzodiazepines are generally an adequate alternative to barbiturates, clinicians can help to minimize the abuse of barbiturates by prescribing them rarely, if ever. In the case of withdrawal reactions, reinstituting and then tapering the offending barbiturate under close clinical supervision can assist the detoxification process.

SECTION TWO:
Hallucinogens

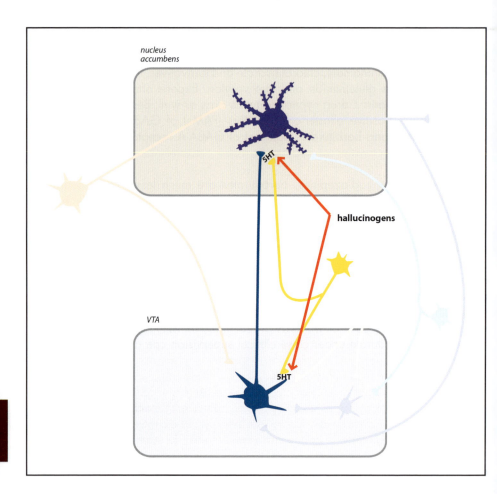

# SECTION TWO:
Hallucinogens (cont'd)

FIGURE 8.2. Hallucinogenic drugs are a group of agents that act at serotonin synapses within the VTA and the nucleus accumbens. These agents produce intoxication, sometimes called a "trip," that is associated with changes in sensory experiences, including visual illusions and hallucinations and an enhanced awareness of both external and internal stimuli and thoughts. These hallucinations are produced with a clear level of consciousness and a lack of confusion and may be both psychedelic (heightened sensory awareness and the subjective experience that one's mind is being expanded) and psychotomimetic (superficially mimicking a state of psychosis).

Specific symptoms of hallucinogen intoxication include visual "trails," in which the image smears into streaks as it moves across a visual trail, macropsia and micropsia, emotional and mood lability, subjective slowing of time, the sense that colors are heard and sounds are seen, intensification of sound perception, and depersonalization and derealization. Other symptoms may include impaired judgment, fear of losing one's mind, anxiety, nausea, tachycardia, increased blood pressure, and increased body temperature. Not surprisingly, hallucinogen intoxication can cause what is perceived as a panic attack, which is often called a "bad trip." As intoxication escalates, one can experience an acute state of disorientation and agitation. This can evolve further into frank psychosis, with delusions and paranoia.

There are 2 major classes of hallucinogenic drugs. The agents in the first class resemble serotonin and include the classic hallucinogens LSD (d-lysergic acid diethylamide), psilocybin, and dimethyltryptamine (DMT). The agents in the second class resemble norepinephrine and dopamine and are related to amphetamine; they include mescaline and DOM (2,5-dimethoxy-4-methylamphetamine). Recently, synthetic chemists have come up with some new "designer drugs," such as MDMA (3,4-methylenedioxymethamphetamine) and "foxy" (5-methoxydiisopropyltryptamine). These are either stimulants or hallucinogens and produce a complex subjective state sometimes referred to as "ecstasy," which is also what abusers call MDMA itself. MDMA produces euphoria, disorientation, confusion, enhanced sociability, and a sense of increased empathy and personal insight.

Hallucinogenic Mechanism and Long-Term Effects

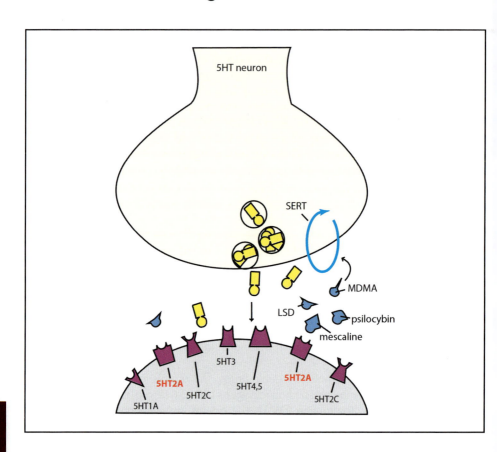

Hallucinogenic Mechanism and Long-Term Effects (cont'd)

FIGURE 8.3. Hallucinogenic drugs are all partial agonists at 5HT2A receptors, which leads to dopamine release. Hallucinogens may have additional actions at other serotonin receptors, particularly 5HT1A and 5HT2C. In particular, MDMA blocks the serotonin transporter (SERT). However, stimulation of 5HT2A receptors seems to be the primary mechanism by which these agents exert their effects.

Hallucinogens can produce incredible tolerance, sometimes after a single dose. Desensitization of 5HT2A receptors is hypothesized to underlie this rapid clinical and pharmacological tolerance. Another unique dimension of hallucinogen abuse is the production of "flashbacks." A flashback is the spontaneous recurrence of some of the symptoms of intoxication that lasts from a few seconds to several hours and occurs in the absence of recent hallucinogen use. This occurs days to months after the last drug experience and can apparently be precipitated by a number of environmental stimuli. The psychopharmacological mechanism underlying flashbacks is unknown, but its phenomenology suggests the possibility of a neurochemical adaptation of the serotonin system that is related to long-lasting reverse tolerance. Alternatively, flashbacks could be a form of emotional conditioning embedded in the amygdala and then triggered when an emotional experience revives the memory of acute intoxication. This is analogous to the types of reexperiencing flashbacks that occur without drugs in patients with posttraumatic stress disorder.

SECTION THREE:
Club Drugs

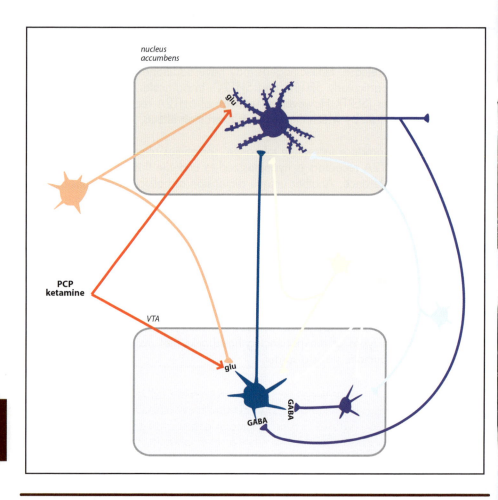

FIGURE 8.4. Phencyclidine (PCP) and ketamine are both considered "club drugs." These agents have actions at glutamate synapses within the reward system.

Club Drugs:
Mechanism and Effects

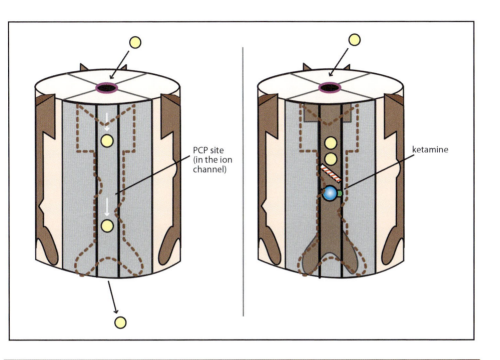

FIGURE 8.5. PCP and ketamine both act as antagonists of NMDA receptors, binding to a site in the calcium channel. Both were originally developed as anesthetics, but PCP proved to be unacceptable for this use because it induces a unique psychotomimetic/hallucinatory experience that is similar to schizophrenia. The NMDA receptor hypoactivity that is caused by PCP has become a model for the same neurotransmitter abnormalities postulated to underlie schizophrenia. Its structurally and mechanism-related analog ketamine causes far less of the psychotomimetic/hallucinatory experience and is still used as an anesthetic. Nevertheless, some people do abuse ketamine.

PCP causes intense analgesia, amnesia, and delirium, stimulant as well as depressant actions, staggering gait, slurred speech, and a unique form of nystagmus (i.e., vertical nystagmus). Higher degrees of intoxication can cause catatonia (excitement alternating with stupor and catalepsy), hallucinations, delusions, paranoia, disorientation, and poor judgment. Overdose can cause coma, extremely high temperature, seizures, and muscle breakdown (rhabdomyolysis).

SECTION FOUR:
Trends in Methods for Getting High

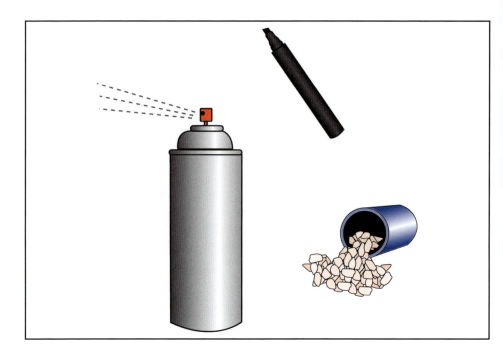

SECTION FOUR:
Trends in Methods for Getting High (cont'd)

FIGURE 8.6. Novel methods for getting high are constantly being sought, from new designer drugs to the misuse of regular household items. Some of the most common current trends for getting high include the use of synthetic stimulants ("bath salts") and huffing.

Bath salts are synthetic stimulants that commonly include the active ingredient methylenedioxypyrovalerone (MDPV) but may contain mephedrone or methylone instead. They are also called plant food and have been sold in mini-marts and smoke shops under names such as Ivory Wave, Purple Wave, and Vanilla Sky. Like other illicit stimulants, bath salts can have reinforcing effects but can also cause agitation, paranoia, hallucinations, suicidality, and chest pain. Suicidality may last even after the stimulatory effects of the drug have worn off. It can be difficult to know if an individual has taken bath salts because these agents do not show up on drug tests.

Until recently, bath salts were unregulated because they were marketed as bath salts and labeled "not for human consumption." On September 7, 2001, however, the United States DEA invoked its "emergency scheduling authority," designating mephedrone, MDPV, and methylone as Schedule I substances and temporarily making it an offence to possess and sell products that contain them. The DEA is evaluating whether to permanently control these agents.

Another common trend is huffing, whereby the fumes of substances such as paint thinner, felt tip markers, glue, and aerosol sprays are inhaled to produce a high. Most recently, there has been an increase in huffing freon, which is found in air conditioners. Huffing can cause a feeling similar to alcohol intoxication, with dizziness, lightheadedness, and disinhibition; it can also cause impaired judgment and possibly hallucinations. Long-term huffing can cause depression, weight loss, and brain damage. Huffing can also be dangerous in the short term, as it can cause sudden death due to cardiac arrest, aspiration, or suffocation. Freon in particular can cause these effects and can also freeze the lungs, making it extremely dangerous. Substances that are huffed do not show up on drug tests.

Stahl's Illustrated | Chapter 9

Psychosocial Treatment for Substance Use Disorders

Psychosocial treatments are an extremely important component of substance use disorder management. Several different methods can be used, depending on the substance of abuse as well as the particular needs of the patient. In addition, psychosocial therapies can be applied in either an individual or a group setting. This chapter covers the most commonly used and recommended psychosocial therapies for patients with substance use disorders.

Psychosocial Treatment for Substance Use Disorders:
Summary

		CBT	MET	Behavioral therapy	IPT	Family therapy	Self-help/ 12-step
Substance of Abuse	Alcohol	X	X	X		X	X
	Opioid	X		X		X	X
	Nicotine	X	X	X			
	Stimulant	X		X			X
	THC		X	X			

CBT: cognitive behavioral therapy. MET: motivational enhancement therapy. Behavioral therapy: contingency management, community reinforcement, cue exposure and relaxation, aversion therapy. IPT: interpersonal therapy. THC: delta-9-tetrahydrocannabinol.

TABLE 9.1. Many of the same general strategies are used to treat addiction to/dependence on different substances of abuse, as shown here. These strategies are described in more detail in Figures 9.1 through 9.6.

Cognitive Behavioral Therapy

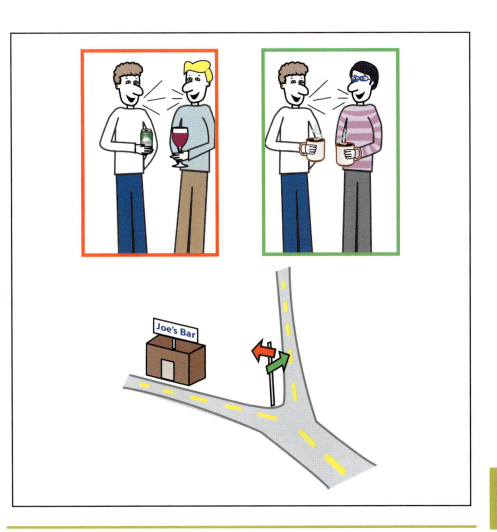

FIGURE 9.1. Cognitive behavioral therapy (CBT) is based on the premise that our behaviors stem from our thoughts and beliefs and therefore that negative thoughts can lead to maladaptive behavior. CBT is designed to modify the behaviors and thoughts/beliefs that contribute to substance abuse and dependence. CBT helps patients identify triggers for substance use, such as particular people or places or even emotions, and helps them develop techniques to either avoid those triggers or to cope with them.

Behavioral Therapy

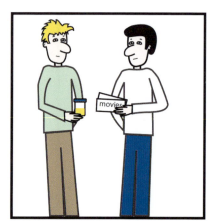

Contingency Management

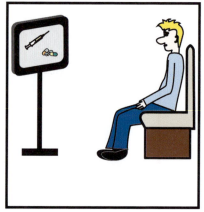

Cue Exposure

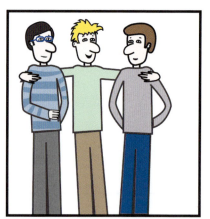

Community Reinforcement

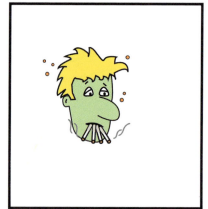

Aversion Therapy

Behavioral Therapy (cont'd)

FIGURE 9.2. Behavioral therapies are intended to help patients unlearn harmful behaviors (e.g., excessive substance use) and learn alternate behaviors (e.g., attending therapy sessions). There are 4 major types of behavioral therapy used for substance use disorders: contingency management, community reinforcement, cue exposure and relaxation, and aversion therapy.

Contingency management has been used with a number of different substances of abuse. It involves incentives for desired behaviors (e.g., attending therapy sessions, adhering to pharmacological treatment) as well as negative consequences for undesirable behaviors (e.g., positive urine sample). Incentives may include vouchers for agreed-upon items.

Community reinforcement is designed to reward patients with substance use disorders for engaging in positive sober activities, such as family and social events. Specifically, the aim is to help create or enhance positive environmental factors that reinforce sobriety. Family and friend involvement is therefore an integral component of this therapy. Treatment may include marriage counseling, job counseling or training, or introduction to substance-free social environments.

With cue exposure, patients are exposed to stimuli that induce craving and drug anticipation but are prevented from actually obtaining the substance, with the idea that this will ultimately lead to the extinction of the conditioned craving response. Relaxation training may be incorporated to help aid the process.

Aversion therapy is intended to eliminate substance use behaviors by associating them with an unpleasant situation (e.g., smoking to the point of illness).

Motivational Enhancement Therapy

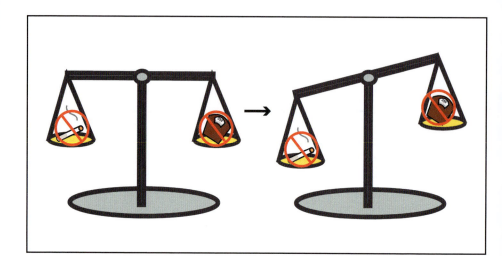

FIGURE 9.3. Motivational interviewing is patient-focused counseling with the direct goal of enhancing one's motivation to change by helping explore and resolve ambivalence (e.g., "I want to stop smoking, but I'm afraid I'll gain weight"). Although it was originally developed to help individuals with problem drinking, it can be used in the treatment of patients with other forms of substance abuse and dependence. In motivational interviewing, the clinician is a facilitator, helping the patient identify, articulate, and resolve his or her own ambivalence without direct persuasion, confrontation, or coercion.

Motivational enhancement therapy (MET) is an adaptation of motivational interviewing whereby the therapist uses feedback to strengthen the patient's own motivation and commitment to change.

Interpersonal Therapy

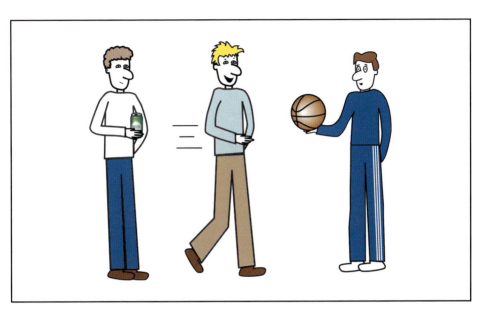

FIGURE 9.4. Interpersonal therapy is used for patients whose substance use disorder may be related to interpersonal conflicts. The aim is for patients to identify dysfunctional relationships and work toward building a new social network that is conducive to a sober lifestyle.

Family Therapy

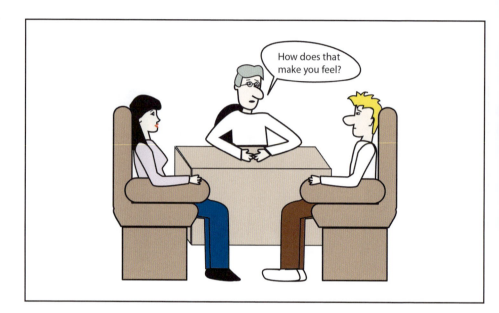

FIGURE 9.5. Family therapy both provides additional information about the patient (e.g., treatment adherence, social adjustment, interaction with substance-using peers) and encourages familial support of abstinence. It can also help improve family relationships. Family therapy may improve adherence to and participation in other forms of therapy as well. This may be a particularly important therapy for adolescents with a substance use disorder.

12-Step Facilitation and 12-Step Fellowships

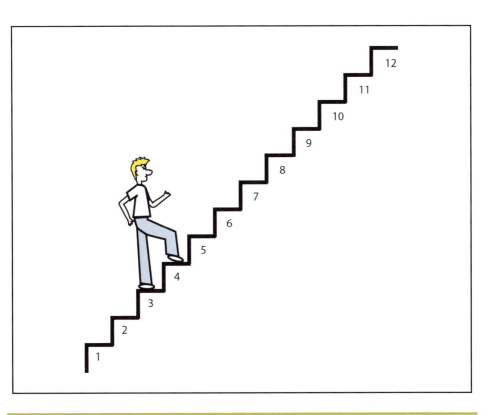

FIGURE 9.6. Twelve-Step Facilitation (TSF) consists of a structured, manual-driven approach to facilitating early recovery from alcohol abuse/alcoholism and other drug abuse/addiction. Its purpose is to help patients accept their need to abstain and actively participate in 12-step fellowships (such as Alcoholics Anonymous, or AA) as a means of maintaining abstinence. It is intended to be implemented on an individual basis in 12–15 sessions and is based on the 12 steps and traditions of AA.

Although mutual support groups such as 12-step fellowships can be very beneficial in helping patients with substance use disorders, these programs are based on the premise that addiction is an illness in which those afflicted are unable to control their use of the drug. As such, they typically require complete abstinence as the goal. This may therefore pose conflict for patients with alcohol use disorder who are attempting to achieve reduced-risk drinking.

Stahl's Illustrated | Chapter 10

Disorders of Impulsivity and Compulsivity

A number of conditions that have been categorized as disorders of impulsivity or compulsivity may be hypothetically linked to abnormal activity of reward circuits, analogous to an addiction. To that end, there has been much interest lately in the potential symptom and neurobiological overlap between substance use disorders, impulse control disorders (ICDs), and obsessive compulsive disorder (OCD). Specifically, a great deal of debate has focused on whether disorders currently classified as ICDs should be considered "behavioral addictions" or obsessive compulsive spectrum disorders, or even whether they qualify as disorders at all. In this chapter, we review both the similarities and differences between substance use disorders and various behavioral addictions/ICDs.

SUDs vs. ICDs

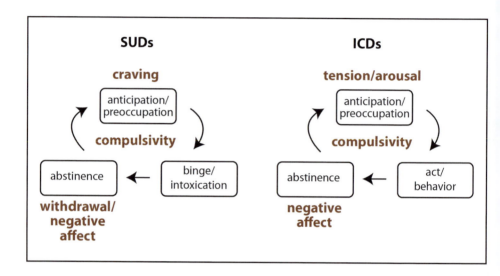

FIGURE 10.1. In Chapter 1, we described drug addiction as a disorder of impulsivity and compulsivity wherein initial, impulsive drug use progresses to compulsive use driven by a desire to reduce the distressing symptoms of withdrawal (left).

This conceptualization has obvious similarities to many disorders that have been considered ICDs (e.g., pathological gambling). That is, individuals with these disorders experience tension and arousal in anticipation of performing the behavior and dysphoric mood (but no physiological withdrawal) when prevented from performing the behavior (right). In addition, the pleasure and gratification that they initially experience when performing the behavior seems to diminish over time, perhaps requiring increasing "doses" (e.g., gambling higher dollar amounts) in order to achieve the same effects (akin to tolerance).

DSM Criteria for SUDs:
Applicable to ICDs?

Maladaptive pattern of substance use leading to significant impairment/distress
(2 or more of the following within 12 months; 2–3 = moderate, >3=severe)

- Recurrent use leading to failure to fulfill major obligations
- Recurrent use in hazardous situations
- Continued use despite persistent or recurrent social problems caused or exacerbated by effects of substance
- Tolerance
- Withdrawal
- Taken in larger amounts or for longer periods than intended
- Persistent desire or unsuccessful efforts to control, reduce, or stop
- Great deal of time spent obtaining, using, or recovering
- Important activities given up or reduced because of substance use
- Continued use despite knowledge of physical or psychological problem likely caused or exacerbated by substance
- Craving or urge to use substance

FIGURE 10.2. The similarities between SUDs and ICDs are also apparent in the diagnostic criteria for substance use disorders. Many ICDs are characterized by continued use despite adverse consequences, craving prior to the behavior, withdrawal (though not physiological) during abstinence, tolerance, and unsuccessful efforts to stop.

Other common features between SUDs and ICDs include early age of onset, overlapping neurobiology (in particular, evidence of involvement of the VTA and the nucleus accumbens as well as dopamine, serotonin, glutamate, and opioids), a possible genetic relationship (supported by a small number of controlled family studies), and response to some of the same treatments (naltrexone, suggesting mu opioid involvement; N-acetylcysteine (NAC), suggesting glutamate involvement). There are also high rates of co-occurrence between various SUDs and ICDs.

Proposed DSM-5 Categorization of Impulsive/Compulsive Disorders

Substance Use and Addictive Disorders	Disruptive, Impulse Control, and Conduct Disorders	Sexual Disorders	Obsessive Compulsive and Related Disorders
Gambling disorder	Pyromania	Hypersexual disorder	Hair pulling (trichotillomania)
	Kleptomania		Skin picking
	Intermittent explosive disorder		

TABLE 10.1. Although there is some evidence in support of the concept of behavioral addiction, controversy remains as to whether the evidence is strong enough to warrant categorizing certain behaviors as addictions. This debate is particularly apparent as experts work to develop DSM-5. Possible categories suggested for the ICDs have been "behavioral and substance addictions" and "impulsive-compulsive disorders." There has also been consideration of including some ICDs in a category with OCD due to some apparent similarities.

As of the time of this writing, currently proposed revisions to the DSM with respect to SUDs and ICDs include:

1. Moving pathological gambling (renamed gambling disorder) from ICDs to "substance use and addictive disorders"
2. Moving pyromania, kleptomania, and intermittent explosive disorder (IED) from ICDs to "disruptive, impulse control, and conduct disorders"
3. Including hypersexual disorder as a "sexual disorder"
4. Moving trichotillomania (renamed hair pulling disorder) to "obsessive compulsive and related disorders"
5. Adding skin picking as a disorder in the "obsessive compulsive and related disorders" category

Other impulsive behaviors have been considered but not recommended for inclusion in DSM-5. These include compulsive shopping, excessive tanning, computer/video game playing, Internet addiction, and food addiction.

Gambling Disorder

> Maladaptive gambling behavior as indicated by 5 or more of the following:
>
> - Preoccupation with gambling
> - Need to gamble with increasing amounts of money to achieve desired excitement
> - Unsuccessful efforts to control, reduce, or stop gambling
> - Restless or irritable when attempting to control, reduce, or stop gambling
> - Gamble to escape from problems or relieve dysphoric mood
> - After losing money gambling, often return another day to get even ("chase" losses)
> - Lie or attempt to conceal extent of gambling
> - Jeopardized or lost a significant relationship or opportunity because of gambling
> - Rely on others to provide money to relieve financial situation caused by gambling

FIGURE 10.3. Pathological gambling has been included as an ICD in the DSM since 1980. Now, in DSM-5, it is proposed that it be renamed gambling disorder and moved to the category Substance Use and Addictive Disorders, making it the only non-substance disorder in that category.

It is obvious from the diagnostic criteria for gambling disorder (which will remain the same except for the removal of the item regarding illegal acts) that there are strong similarities between SUDs and pathological gambling. This is based on data showing that pathological gambling involves repeated unsuccessful efforts to stop or cut back, psychological withdrawal (irritability, restlessness) when not gambling, tolerance (gambling higher and higher dollar amounts), and diminished ability to resist the impulse to gamble despite adverse consequences.

Treatment studies for pathological gambling suggest a mechanistic relationship to SUDs. The strongest data are for the mu opioid receptor antagonists naltrexone and nalmefene. There is also a positive study of lithium in patients with comorbid bipolar disorder. Antipsychotics have not demonstrated efficacy, and data for SSRIs are mixed. Psychosocial treatments, including CBT, MET, and 12-step programs, are also beneficial.

Pyromania and Kleptomania

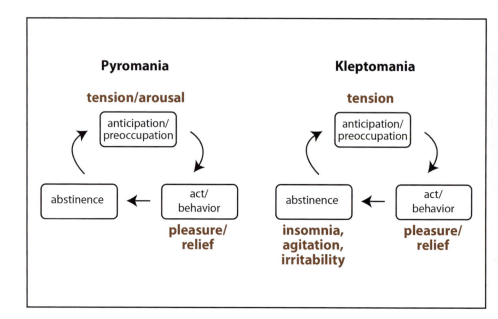

FIGURE 10.4. Pyromania and kleptomania are currently categorized as ICDs, and proposed revisions for DSM-5 will continue to include them as disorders of impulse control. Both of these disorders involve tension and/or arousal prior to committing the act, relief or pleasure following the act, and (though not part of the formal criteria) discomfort when attempting to stop the behavior. Thus, there are parallels to substance use disorders. However, neither disorder has been extensively studied, and the association between them and SUDs is somewhat theoretical at this point. Naltrexone has demonstrated preliminary efficacy in the treatment of kleptomania, and there is evidence that CBT is effective as well.

Intermittent Explosive Disorder and Impulsive Aggression

Intermittent Explosive Disorder

Severe discrete episodes of failure to resist aggressive impulses that result in serious assaultive acts or destruction of property

Degree of aggressiveness expressed is grossly out of proportion to any precipitating psychosocial stressors

Aggressive episodes are not better accounted for by another mental disorder or a general medical condition and are not due to the direct physiological effects of a substance

---

FIGURE 10.5. Like pyromania and kleptomania, intermittent explosive disorder will likely continue to be classified as an ICD. Intermittent explosive disorder is characterized by the failure to resist aggressive impulses that result in serious assault or destruction of property. The aggression is disproportionate to any provocation, is not premeditated, and is not accounted for by another condition or the direct effects of a substance.

Impulsive aggression is precipitated by a trigger, usually a stressor that invokes negative emotions, and involves high levels of autonomic arousal. There is no evidence of a progression from impulsivity to compulsivity with intermittent explosive disorder or with impulsive aggression in general, and it is not considered an addictive disorder. There is, however, an indirect relationship between impulsive aggression and substance use, as drug intoxication and addiction substantially increase the risk for this behavior. Although impulsive aggression is not directly regulated by the reward system, what is known about its neurobiology suggests that there are overlaps and that the alterations that occur with addiction may confer greater risk for impulsive aggression.

Impulsive Aggression

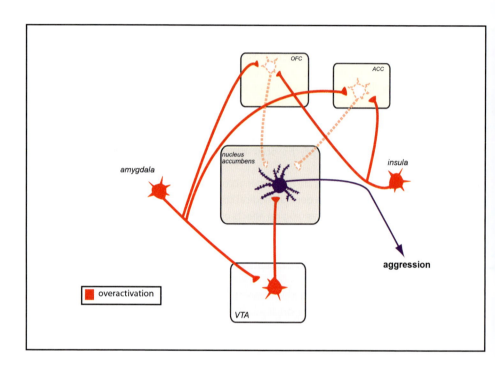

Impulsive Aggression (cont'd)

FIGURE 10.6. From a neurobiological perspective, pathological impulsive aggression seems to occur when there is an imbalance between "bottom up" signals coming from the amygdala and the insula and "top down" controls coming from the orbital frontal cortex (OFC) and the anterior cingulate cortex (ACC). That is, the amygdala and insula interpret incoming stimuli in relation to past emotional conditioning encoded in the amygdala and use that information to trigger "drives." The orbital frontal and anterior cingulate cortices in turn regulate the reaction to these drives based on an assessment of reward and punishment. Various neuromodulators regulate these brain regions, including serotonin, norepinephrine, dopamine, GABA, glutamate, acetylcholine, and neuropeptides. Of these, serotonin is the most strongly implicated in the regulation of aggression.

Imbalance in the bottom up/top down brain circuitry may occur due to hypoactivity of the prefrontal cortex and/or hyperactivity of limbic regions, as is seen in drug addiction. It is therefore not surprising that drug intoxication and addiction increase the risk for impulsive aggression. In fact, the presence of drug abuse, psychosis, and a personality disorder is the worst combination in terms of risk for impulsive aggression.

Although there is limited direct research on the effects of treatment for aggression, there are some data to suggest the efficacy of various psychotropic agents, supported by theoretical neurobiological mechanisms. Serotonin reuptake inhibitors may enhance prefrontal inhibition of limbic activity by increasing serotonin availability in the orbital frontal cortex. Anticonvulsant mood stabilizers, many of which affect GABA and/or glutamate neurotransmission, may reduce limbic irritability. Atypical antipsychotics can both decrease subcortical dopaminergic stimulation via dopamine 2 antagonism and increase prefrontal inhibition via serotonin 2A antagonism. Current clinical evidence suggests that clozapine and high doses of atypical antipsychotics may be the most effective treatments for aggression. Other psychotropic agents may also be able to mediate aggression; these include stimulants, which may increase frontal inhibition, and opioids, which may reduce drive.

Hypersexual Disorder

> Over at least 6 months, recurrent and intense sexual fantasies, urges, and behaviors in association with 4 or more of the following:
>
> - Excessive time consumed by sexual fantasies and urges and by planning for and engaging in sexual behavior
> - Repetitive engagement in these sexual fantasies, urges, and behaviors in response to dysphoric mood states
> - Repetitive engagement in these sexual fantasies, urges, and behaviors in response to stressful life events
> - Repetitive but unsuccessful efforts to control or reduce these sexual fantasies, urges, and behaviors
> - Repetitive engagement in sexual behavior while disregarding the risk for physical or emotional harm to self or others
>
> There must be clinically significant personal distress or impairment in important areas of functioning associated with the frequency and intensity of these sexual fantasies, urges, and behaviors

FIGURE 10.7. Hypersexual disorder has been proposed for inclusion in the DSM-5. Variations of hypersexual disorder have existed in the DSM since the third edition, and the disorder has been conceptualized by different experts as an obsessive compulsive disorder, an impulse control disorder, "out of control" sexual behavior, or a sexual addiction. Although the suggested DSM-5 criteria for hypersexual disorder have much in common with the criteria for a substance use disorder, hypersexual disorder is not proposed to be included with addictive disorders but rather with sexual disorders.

Treatment for hypersexual disorder has not been rigorously studied but may include both psychosocial and pharmacological methods. SSRIs, antiandrogens, and CBT have demonstrated efficacy in small trials.

Excessive Internet Use and Other Impulsive/Compulsive Disorders

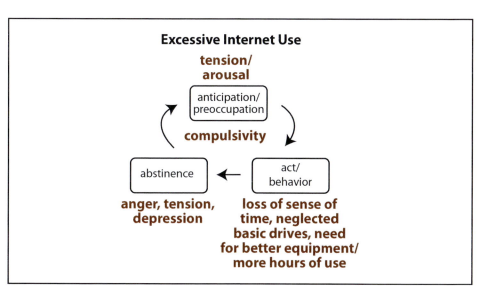

FIGURE 10.8. There are limited data regarding the course, neurobiology, and treatment response for excessive Internet use, and it is not currently recognized as a formal diagnosis. The studies that do exist have methodological differences, including how Internet addiction is defined, that make their results difficult to interpret. Symptoms that have been observed include excessive use associated with loss of time or neglect of basic needs; psychological withdrawal characterized by anger, tension, or depression when denied access to a computer; tolerance, indicated by a need for better equipment or more hours of use; and adverse social and occupational effects.

There are no evidence-based treatments for Internet addiction. When it is treated, psychosocial methods such as CBT are generally used.

As with excessive Internet use, there are currently limited data regarding computer/video game addiction, compulsive buying, and excessive tanning, and debate continues as to whether these should be classified as addictive disorders, obsessive compulsive spectrum disorders, or something else.

Food Addiction

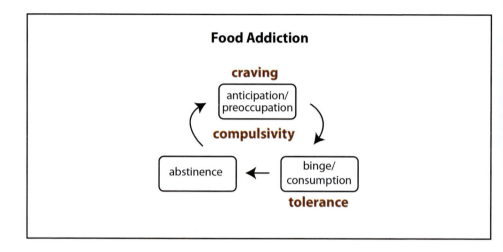

FIGURE 10.9. Like drugs, food has powerful reinforcing effects, and the circuitry that regulates the rewarding effects of drugs overlaps that of the rewarding effects of food. In addition, there is evidence to suggest that the neurobiological changes associated with the progression to compulsive drug use and addiction are also seen in individuals with compulsive eating behaviors. When exposed to food cues, obese individuals exhibit increased activation (compared to lean individuals) in regions that process palatability. In contrast, obese individuals exhibit decreased activation of reward circuits during actual food consumption. This is analogous to cravings and tolerance in patients with SUDs. There is also decreased activation of the prefrontal cortex in patients with obesity, just as in patients with drug addiction, suggesting impairment in the reactive reward system.

Despite evidence suggesting that SUDs and obesity have overlapping neurobiological dysfunction, food addiction is not currently proposed as an addition to DSM-5.

Hair Pulling, Skin Picking, and OCD

Hair Pulling Disorder (Trichotillomania)	Skin Picking Disorder
Recurrent hair pulling resulting in hair loss	Recurrent skin picking resulting in lesions
Hair pulling causes clinically significant distress or functional impairment	Skin picking causes clinically significant distress or functional impairment
Hair pulling is not due to direct physiological effects of a substance or medical condition	Skin picking is not due to direct physiological effects of a substance or medical condition
Hair pulling is not restriced to symptoms of another mental disorder	Skin picking is not restriced to symptoms of another mental disorder

FIGURE 10.10. Trichotillomania is classified with impulse control disorders in the DSM-IV-TR; however, recent work in the development of the DSM-5 has led to the recommendation that it be moved to a category called "obsessive-compulsive and related disorders." It is also recommended that criteria B (increasing tension before pulling hair) and C (pleasure or relief when pulling hair) be removed, as clinical data do not support the diagnostic utility of these criteria. That is, although these symptoms do occur in many patients with trichotillomania, not all patients experience them, and individuals with trichotillomania are not distinguishable based on them.

Skin picking, which would have fallen under ICDs not elsewhere classified in the DSM-IV-TR, is recommended to be included in obsessive-compulsive and related disorders, with criteria that parallel those for hair pulling disorder (trichotillomania).

Stahl's Illustrated

Summary

- A substance use disorder can be conceptualized as a progression from an impulsive to a compulsive disorder

- This progression is linked to alterations not only in dopamine and the reward circuit, but also in other neurotransmitters and circuits involved in memory, motivation, executive function, and stress

- Of particular importance is the opioid system, which mediates the hedonic evaluation of natural rewards and also seems to play a role in drug reinforcement for numerous substances

- The management of SUDs can differ by substance, but it generally involves both psychosocial and pharmacological treatment

- The substances with evidence-based pharmacological treatments are alcohol, nicotine, and opioids

- Although there is some evidence in support of the concept of behavioral addiction, controversy remains as to whether the evidence is strong enough to warrant categorizing certain behaviors as addictions

- Currently, only pathological gambling is being recategorized as an addictive disorder

Stahl's Illustrated Abbreviations

5HT	serotonin	mGluR	metabotropic glutamate receptor
ACC	anterior cingulate cortex		
ACh	acetylcholine	MOR	mu opioid receptor
AMPA	alpha amino-3-hydroxy-5-methyl-4-isoxazolepropionic acid	NAc	nucleus accumbens
		NE	norepinephrine
		NMDA	N-methyl-d-aspartate
BZ	benzodiazepine	NPY	neuropeptide Y
CB	cannabinoid	OCD	obsessive compulsive disorder
CBT	cognitive behavioral therapy		
		OFC	orbitofrontal cortex
CRF	corticotropin releasing factor	PCP	phencyclidine
		PFC	prefrontal cortex
DA	dopamine	POMC	pro-opiomelanocortin
DLPFC	dorsolateral prefrontal cortex	PPT/LDT	pedunculopontine and laterodorsal tegmental nucleus
DMT	dimethyltryptamine		
DSM	*Diagnostic and Statistical Manual of Mental Disorders*	SERT	serotonin transporter
		SSRI	selective serotonin reuptake inhibitor
Dyn	dynorphin	SUD	substance use disorder
EC	endocannabinoid	TCA	tricyclic antidepressant
GABA	gamma aminobutyric acid	THC	delta-9-tetrahydrocannabinol
glu	glutamate		
ICD	impulse control disorder	VMAT	vesicular monoamine transporter
IED	intermittent explosive disorder		
		VMPFC	ventromedial prefrontal cortex
IPT	interpersonal therapy		
LC	locus coeruleus	VSCC	voltage-sensitive calcium channel
LSD	d-lysergic acid diethylamide		
		VTA	ventral tegmental area
LTP	long-term potentiation		
MDMA	3,4-methylenedioxymethamphetamine		
MET	motivational enhancement therapy		

Stahl's Illustrated

References

Alvarez Y, Farre M, Fonseca F, Torrens M. Anticonvulsant drugs in cocaine dependence: a systematic review and meta-analysis. J Subst Abuse Treatment 2010;38(1):66-73.

Amato L, Minozzi S, Pani PP et al. Dopamine agonists for the treatment of cocaine dependence. Cochrane Database Syst Rev 2011;12:CD003352.

Ambrogne JA. Reduced-risk drinking as a treatment goal: what clinicians need to know. J Subst Abuse Treatment 2002;22(1):45-53.

American Psychiatric Association. Practice guideline for the treatment of patients with substance use disorders, second edition. Am J Psychiatry 2007;164(4):1-86.

Aolanki DR, Koyyalagunta D, Shah RV, Silverman S, Manchikanti L. Monitoring opioid adherence in chronic pain patients: assessment of risk of substance issues. Pain Physician 2011;14:E119-31.

Bowden-Jones H, Clark L. Pathological gambling: a neurobiological and clinical update. Br J Psychiatry 2011;199:87-9.

Chen BT, Hopf FW, Bonci A. Synaptic plasticity in the mesolimbic system: therapeutic implications for substance abuse. Ann NY Acad Sci 2010;1187:129-39.

Coccaro EF. Intermittent explosive disorder: development of integrated research criteria for Diagnostic and Statistical Manual of Mental Disorders, Fifth Edition. Compr Psychiatry 2011;52(2):119-25.

Collins GT, Narasimhan D, Cunningham AR et al. Long-lasting effects of a PEGylated mutant cocaine esterase (CocE) on the reinforcing and discriminative stimulus effects of cocaine in rats. Neuropsychopharmacology 2012;37(5):1092-103.

Crane R. The most addictive drug, the most deadly substance: smoking cessation tactics for the busy clinician. Prim Care Clin Office Pract 2007;34:117-35.

Czoty PW, Roberts DSC. Thinking outside the synapse: pharmacokinetic based medications for cocaine addiction. Neuropsychopharmacology 2012;37:1079-80.

Dalley JW, Everitt BJ, Robbins TW. Impulsivity, compulsivity, and top-down cognitive control. Neuron 2011;69:680-94.

Deadwyler SA. Electrophysiological correlates of abused drugs: relation to natural rewards. Ann NY Acad Sci 2010;1187:140-7.

Dodrill CL, Helmer DA, Kosten TR. Prescription pain medication dependence. Am J Psychiatry 2011;168(5):466-71.

Ebbert JO, Croghan IT, Sood A, Schroeder DR, Hays JT, Hurt RD. Varenicline and bupropion sustained-release combination therapy for smoking cessation. Nicotine Tobacco Res 2009;11(3):234-9.

Edens E, Massa A, Petrakis I. Novel pharmacological approaches to drug abuse treatment. Curr Top Behav Neurosci 2010;3:343-86.

el-Guebaly N, Mudry T, Zohar J, Tavares H, Potenza MN. Compulsive features in behavioral addictions: the case of pathological gambling. Addiction 2011;Epub ahead of print.

Everitt BJ, Belin D, Economidou D et al. Neural mechanisms underlying the vulnerability to develop compulsive drug-seeking habits and addiction. Philos Trans Royal Soc B 2008;363:3125-35.

Everitt BJ, Robbins TW. Neural systems of reinforcement for drug addiction: from actions to habits to compulsion. Nat Neurosci 2005;8(11):1481-9.

Feltenstein MW, See RE. The neurocircuitry of addiction: an overview. Br J Pharmacol 2008;154:261-74.

Figee M. Vink M, de Geus F et al. Dysfunctional reward circuitry in obsessive-compulsive disorder. Biol Psychiatry 2011;69:867-74.

Fontenelle LF, Oostermeijer S, Harrison BJ, Pantelis C, Yucel M. Obsessive-compulsive disorder, impulse control disorders and drug addiction: common features and potential treatments. Drugs 2011;71(7):827-40.

Garcia FD, Thibaut F. Sexual addictions. Am J Drug Alcohol Abuse 2010;36:254-60.

George O, Koob GF. Individual differences in prefrontal cortex function and the transition from drug use to drug dependence. Neurosci Biobehav Rev 2010;35:232-47.

Gerrits MAFM, Lesscher HBM, van Ree JM. Drug dependence and the endogenous opioid system. Eur Neuropsychopharmacol 2003;13:424-34.

Goldstein RZ, Volkow ND. Dysfunction of the prefrontal cortex in addiction: neuroimaging findings and clinical implications. Nat Rev Neurosci 2011;12(11):652-69.

Grant JE, Odlaug BL, Kim SW. Kleptomania: clinical characteristics and relationship to substance use disorders. Am J Drug Alcohol Abuse 2010;36:291-5.

Grant JE, Potenza MN, Weinstein A, Gorelick DA. Introduction to behavioral addictions. Am J Drug Alcohol Abuse 2010;36:233-41.

Hays JT, Ebbert JO, Sood A. Treating tobacco dependence in light of the 2008 US Department of Health and Human Services clinical practice guideline. Mayo Clin Proc 2009;84(8):730-5.

Heinz AJ, Beck A, Meyer-Lindenberg A, Sterzer P, Heinz A. Cognitive and neurobiological mechanisms of alcohol-related aggression. Nat Rev Neurosci 2011;12(7):400-13.

Hinic D. Problems with 'internet addiction' diagnosis and classification. Psychiatria Danubina 2011;23(2):145-51.

Jatlow P, Mccance EF, Bradberry CW, Elsworth JD, Taylor JR, Roth RH. Alcohol plus cocaine: the whole is more than the sum of its parts. Ther Drug Monitoring 1996;18(4):460-4.

Kafka MP. Hypersexual disorder: a proposed diagnosis for DSM-V. Arch Sex Behav 2010; 39(2):377–400.

Kalivas PW. The glutamate homeostasis hypothesis of addiction. Nat Rev Neurosci 2009;10:561-72.

Kauer JA, Malenka RC. Synaptic plasticity and addiction. Nat Rev Neurosci 2007;8:844-58.

Koob GF. Dynamics of neuronal circuits in addiction: reward, antireward, and emotional memory. Pharmacopsychiatry 2009;42(suppl 1):S32-41.

Koob GF, Le Moal M. Addiction and the brain antireward system. Annu Rev Psychol 2008;59:29-53.

Koob GF, Simon EJ. The neurobiology of addiction: where we have been and where we are going. J Drug Issues 2009;39(1):115-32.

Koob GF, Volkow ND. Neurocircuitry of addiction. Neuropsychopharmacol 2010;35:217-38.

Kourosh AS, Harrington CR, Adinoff B. Tanning as a behavioral addiction. Am J Drug Alcohol Abuse 2010;36:284-90.

Large M, Sharma S, Compton MT, Slade T, Nielssen O. Cannabis use and earlier onset of psychosis: a systematic meta-analysis. Arch Gen Psychiatry 2011;68(6):555-61.

Lejoyeux M, Weinstein A. Compulsive buying. Am J Drug Alcohol Abuse 2010;36:248-53.

Le Merrer J, Becker JAJ, Befort K, Kieffer BL. Reward processing by the opioid system in the brain. Physiol Rev 2009;89:1379-1412.

Martin-Fardon R, Zorrilla EP, Ciccocioppo R, Weiss F. Role of innate and drug-induced dysregulation of brain stress and arousal systems in addiction: focus on corticotropin-releasing factor, nociceptin/orphanin FQ, and orexin/hypocretin. Brain Res 2010;1314:145-61.

McCance EF, Price LH, Kosten TR, Jatlow PI. Cocaethylene: pharmacology, physiology and behavioral effects in humans. J Pharmacol Exp Ther 1995;274(1):215-23.

McCance-Katz EF, Kosten TR, Jatlow P. Concurrent use of cocaine and alcohol is more potent and potentially more toxic than use of either alone—a multiple dose study. Biol Psychiatry 1998;44(4):250-9.

National Institute on Alcohol Abuse and Alcoholism. Available at: http://www.niaaa.nih.gov.

Nicholls L, Bragaw L, Ruetsch C. Opioid dependence treatment and guidelines. J Managed Care Pharm 2010;16(1-b):S14-21.

Odlaug BL, Grant JE. Pathologic skin picking. Am J Drug Alcohol Abuse 2010;36:296-303.

Pani PP, Trogu E, Vecchi S, Amato L. Antidepressants for cocaine dependence and problematic cocaine use. Cochrane Database Syst Rev 2011;12:CD002950.

Physician's desk reference. Montvale, NJ: Thomson PDR; 2010.

Piper ME, Smith SS, Schlam TR et al. A randomized placebo-controlled clinical trial of 5 smoking cessation pharmacotherapies. Arch Gen Psychiatry 2009;66(11):254-62.

Raupach T, van Schayck CP. Pharmacotherapy for smoking cessation: current advances and research topics. CNS Drugs 2011;5(5):371-82.

Robbins TW, Ersche KD, Everitt BJ. Drug addiction and the memory systems of the brain. Ann NY Acad Sci 2008;1141:1-21.

Ross S, Peselow E. The neurobiology of addictive disorders. Clin Neuropharmacol 2009;32:269-76.

Serrano A, Parsons LH. Endocannabinoid influence in drug reinforcement, dependence and addiction-related behaviors. Pharmacol Ther 2011;132:215-41.

Shah SD, Wilken LA, Winkler SR, Lin SJ. Systematic review and meta-analysis of combination therapy for smoking cessation. J Am Pharm Assoc 2003;48(5):659-65.

Soyka M, Kranzler HR, Berglund M et al. World Federation of Societies of Biological Psychiatry (WFSBP) guidelines for biological treatment of substance use and related disorders, part 1: alcoholism. World J Biol Psychiatry 2008;9(1):6-23.

Stein DJ, Grant JE, Franklin ME et al. Trichotillomania (hair pulling disorder), skin picking disorder, and stereotypic movement disorder: toward DSM-V. Depression Anxiety 2010;27:611-26.

Steinberg MB, Greenhaus S, Schmelzer AC et al. Triple-combination pharmacotherapy for medically ill smokers: a randomized trial. Ann Intern Med 2009;150(7):447-54.

Teter CJ, Falone AE, Bakaian AM et al. Medication adherence and attitudes in patients with bipolar disorder and current versus past substance use disorder. Psychiatry Res 2011;190(2-3):253-8.

Torregrossa MM, Corlett PR, Taylor JR. Aberrant learning and memory in addiction. Neurobiol Learning Memory 2011;96:609-23.

Vandrey R, Haney M. Pharmacotherapy for cannabis dependence: how close are we? CNS Drugs 2009;23(7):543-53.

Veilleux JC, Colvin PJ, Anderson J, York C, Heinz AJ. A review of opioid dependence treatment: pharmacological and psychosocial interventions to treat opioid addiction. Clin Psychol Rev 2010:30:155-66.

Volkow ND, Wang GJ, Fowler JS, Tomasi D, Telang F. Addiction: beyond dopamine reward circuitry. PNAS 2011;108(37):15037-42.

Volkow ND, Wang GJ, Fowler JS, Tomasi D. Addiction circuitry in the human brain. Annu Rev Pharmacol Toxicol 2012;52:321-36.

Volkow ND, Wang GJ, Telang F et al. Cocaine cues and dopamine in dorsal striatum: mechanisms of craving in cocaine addiction. J Neurosci 2006;226(24):6583-8.

Volkow ND, Wang GJ, Fowler JS, Tomasi D, Baler R. Food and drug reward: overlapping circuits in human obesity and addiction. Curr Top Behav Neurosci 2011;Epub ahead of print.

Wareham JD, Potenza MN. Pathological gambling and substance use disorders. Am J Drug Alcohol Abuse 2010;36(5):242-7.

Wee S, Hicks MJ, De BP et al. Novel cocaine vaccine linked to a disrupted adenovirus gene transfer vector blocks cocaine psychostimulant and reinforcing effects. Neuropsychopharmacology 2012;37(5):1083-91.

Weinstein AM. Computer and video game addiction—a comparison between game users and non-game users. Am J Drug Alcohol Abuse 2010;36:268-76.

Weinstein AM, Lejoyeux M. Internet addiction or excessive internet use. Am J Drug Alcohol Abuse 2010;36:277-83.

Wiener SE, Sutijono D, Moon CH, et al. Patients with detectable cocaethylene are more likely to require intensive care unit admission after trauma. Am J Emerg Med 2010;28(9):1051-5.

Willenbring ML, Massey SH, Gardner MB. Helping patients who drink too much: an evidence-based guide for primary care physicians. Am Fam Physician 2009;80(1):44-50.

Wise RA, Morales M. A ventral tegmental CRF-glutamate-dopamine interaction in addiction. Brain Res 2010;1314:38-43.

Stahl's Illustrated

Index

12-step fellowships, 141

aberrant behavior, 2
abstinence, 4, 6–7: acamprosate, 52; disulfiram, 56; familial support, 140; mutual support groups, 141; naltrexone, 54, 73; and reduced-risk drinking, 48–9; smoking, 85, 94; from stimulant use, 109; topiramate, 57
abuse, defined, 2
acamprosate, alcohol abstinence, 52–3
acetylcholine (ACh), 16, 78, 151
acute withdrawal, mechanism of, 30–1
addiction, 1–2: neurobiology of, 24–5; patterns of, 6–7; risk factors for, 5
addiction cycle, 4, 28–9
aggression, impulsive, 149–51
alcohol, 35: consumption and risk of AUD, 41; mechanism of action in the VTA, 36–7; mechanism of dopamine increase, 14; monitoring and follow-up, 60; pattern of addiction, 6–7; pharmacological treatments, 50–7; psychosocial treatment, 51; recommended drinking limits, 40; reduced-risk drinking, 48–9; screening methods, 42–3; standard drink, 38–9; treatment strategies, 44–7; withdrawal syndrome, treatment of, 58–9

alcohol withdrawal syndrome (AWS), treating, 58–9
alpha 4 beta 2 nicotinic receptors, 78–81
amotivational syndrome, long-term marijuana use, 116
AMPA/NMDA receptor ratio, 26–7
amphetamine, 99–103
amygdala: CRF activation during acute withdrawal, 30–1; and flashbacks, 127; impulsive aggression, 150–1; role in reward system, 18–19, 23; stress circuit, 28–9
anterior cingulate cortex (ACC), 25, 151
anticonvulsants, 57, 107, 151
antidepressants, 9, 50, 65, 75, 107
atypical antipsychotics, aggression, 151
AUDIT (Alcohol Use Disorders Identification Test), 42–3
aversion therapy, 136–7

barbiturates, 123
"bath salts," 131
behavioral addictions *see* impulse control disorders (ICDs)
behavioral therapies, 136–7
benzodiazepines (BZs): for alcohol withdrawal, 50, 59; alternative to barbiturates, 123; for opioid withdrawal, 75

brain stress system, 28–9
brief intervention for smoking cessation, 83
buprenorphine, 70–1: DEA DATA 2000 waiver to prescribe, 72; opioid withdrawal treatment, 65, 67, 74–5
bupropion, smoking cessation, 85, 94–5

cannabinoids (CBs), 16–17: actions on reward circuits, 114; mechanism of dopamine increase, 14; retrograde neurotransmitters, 115
clonidine/naltrexone, 74–5
clonidine, opioid withdrawal, 74–5
club drugs, 128–9
cocaethylene, 106
cocaine, 99–100: effects and treatment, 105; and ethanol interaction, cocaethylene, 106; experimental treatments, 110–11; pharmacological treatment, 107; progression of abuse, 104; route of administration, 103; vs. methamphetamine, 101–2; withdrawal symptoms, 109
cocaine esterase (CocE), 111
cognitive behavioral therapy (CBT), 135–6
community reinforcement, 136–7
comorbid psychiatric illness and substance use, treatment issues, 8–9
compulsion/compulsivity, 4, 6: categorization of disorders of, 146; drug addiction as disorder of, 4, 144; neurobiology of, 24–5; obsessive compulsive disorder, 143, 146, 155; stress circuit implicated in, 28–9
conditioning, 23, 56, 104, 127, 151
contingency management, 136–7
corticotropin releasing factor (CRF), 28–31, 33
craving, 4, 6, 7, 23–5, 144: bupropion alleviating, 94; cue exposure therapy, 137; methadone suppressing, 69; nicotine patches controling, 90

cue exposure, 136–7

delta-9-tetrahydrocannabinol (THC), 114, 119
delta opioid receptors, 63
dependence, defined, 2
"designer drugs," 125
diagnostic criteria *see* DSM-V proposed criteria
dimethyltryptamine (DMT), 125
disorders of impulsivity and compulsivity, 143: gambling disorder, 147; hair pulling, skin picking and OCD, 155; hypersexual disorder, 152; impulsive aggression and IED, 149; proposed DSM-5 categorization of, 146; pyromania and kleptomania, 148; similarities between SUDs and ICDs, 144–5
disulfiram, alcohol abstinence, 56
dopamine (DA) and reward circuit, 12–18: actions of alcohol, 36–7, 54; actions of nicotine, 78–81, 94; actions of opioids, 62; and compulsive use/addiction, 25; conditioning mechanism, 23; and stimulant abuse, 100–4; tolerance and acute withdrawal, 30–1
dopamine transporter (DAT), 14, 101–2
dorsal striatum, 13, 23–5
dorsolateral prefrontal cortex (DLPFC), 13, 19, 21, 25
drinking behavior and risk of AUD, 41
drinking limits, 40
dronabinol, marijuana withdrawal, 119
drug administration route, 82, 103
DSM criteria for SUDs, similarities to ICDs, 145
DSM-V proposed criteria: hair pulling and skin picking, 155; hypersexual disorder, 152; for ICDs, 146, 155; for SUDs, 3, 146
dynorphin (Dyn), 30–2, 63
dysphoria, 6, 7, 32, 63–4, 144

"ecstasy," 125
endocannabinoids, 115
endogenous opioids, 49, 54, 62–3
enkephalin, 28, 36–7, 62–3
epigenetic mechanisms, 5, 33
exogenous opioids, 63

family therapy, 140
flashbacks, hallucinogen abuse, 127
follow-up: alcohol use disorder, 60; opioid withdrawal, 67; smoking cessation, 84
food addiction, 154
"foxy" (5-methoxydiisopropyltryptamine), 125
freon, "huffing" of, 131

GABA (gamma aminobutyric acid), 14, 16–19, 22–3: acamprosate effects, 52; alcohol effects, 36–7; and anxiety/panic attacks in MWS, 32; nicotine effects, 78–9; role in tolerance and acute withdrawal, 30–1; sedative hypnotics, 122–3; topiramate effects, 57
gambling disorder, 147
genetic contributions to addiction, 5
glutamate (glu), 16, 30: acamprosate effects on, 52; action of club drugs, 128; and acute withdrawal, 31; and alcohol action in the VTA, 36–7; and development of addiction, 26–7; and nicotine action in the VTA, 78–9; topiramate's effects on, 57
goal-directed behavior, output of reward system, 22
gum, nicotine replacement therapy, 88–9

hair pulling disorder, 146, 155
hallucinogens, 124–5: long-term effects, 127; mechanism of action, 126–7
huffing, 131
hypersexual disorder, 152

impulse control disorders (ICDs), 143: criteria for SUBs applicable to, 145; food addiction, 154; intermittent explosive disorder (IED), 149; Internet addiction, 153; pathological gambling, 147; proposed DSM-5 categorization of, 146; pyromania and kleptomania, 148; versus SUDs, 144
impulsion/impulsivity: brain circuits implicated in, 28–9; impulsive aggression, 149–51; progression to compulsivity, 4
impulsive aggression, 149–51
intermittent explosive disorder (IED), 149
Internet addiction, 153
interpersonal therapy (IPT), 139
intoxication, 4, 6, 7: effects of phencyclidine (PCP), 129; symptoms of hallucinogenic, 125; symptoms of marijuana, 116; symptoms of opioid, 64; treatment of stimulant, 105
irritability, 7, 32, 75, 105, 119, 151

kappa opioid receptors, 63
ketamine, 128–9
kleptomania, 148

long-term potentiation (LTP), 27
lozenges, nicotine replacement therapy, 88, 93
LSD (D-lysergic acid diethylamide), 125

marijuana, 7, 113: actions on reward circuits, 114; effects of, 116; pattern of addiction, 6–7; pharmacological treatment, 117; psychosocial treatment, 118; and retrograde neurotransmission, 115; withdrawal symptoms, 119
MDMA (3,4-methylene-dioxymethamphetamine), 125, 127
mephedrone in "bath salts," 131
mesolimbic dopamine pathway, 12–13

metabotropic glutamate receptor (mGluR), 36–7
methadone, 65, 67–9, 74–5
methamphetamine, 99–105, 109
methylenedioxypyrovalerone (MDPV), 131
methylone in "bath salts", 131
methylphenidate, 99–103
misuse, defined, 2
monitoring of AUD patients, 60
motivational enhancement therapy (MET), 138
motivational interviewing, 138
motivational withdrawal syndrome (MWS), 32
mu opioid receptor (MOR), 14, 16: actions of alcohol, 36–7, 54; buprenorphine, 70; methadone, 69; naloxone, 71; naltrexone, 54, 73; reinforcement role, 63
multiple substance use, 9, 27

N-methyl-D-aspartate (NMDA), 26–7, 36–7, 52, 129
naloxone, 71, 75
naltrexone: for alcohol use disorder, 54–5; kleptomania treatment, 148; for opioid use disorder, 67, 73; opioid withdrawal treatment, 74–5
nasal inhalers, 88, 92
nasal sprays, 88, 91
National Institute on Alcohol Abuse and Alcoholism (NIAAA), 40–1, 43
neurobiology of reward and drug addiction, 11: acute withdrawal, 30–1; addiction cycle and brain stress system, 28–9; compulsive use/addiction, 24–5; conditioning to reward cues, 23; dopamine and reward, 12–15; goal-directed behavior, turning reward into, 22; loss of control over drug use, 26–7; motivational withdrawal syndrome (MWS), 32; neurotransmitter regulation of mesolimbic reward, 16; reactive reward system, 18; reflective reward system, 19; relapse, 33; substrates for reinforcing effects of drugs, 17; temptation vs. willpower, 20–1; tolerance development, 30–1
neuropeptide Y (NPY), 30–2
neurotransmitters, 16, 17, 30–1: endocannabinoids as retrograde, 115; endogenous opioid, 63; involved in symptoms of MWS, 32
nicotine, 77: actions in the VTA, 78–9; alpha 4 beta 2 nicotine receptors, 80–1; brief intervention for smoking cessation, 83; dopamine increase, mechanism of, 14; effects of, function of delivery mode, 82; management strategy, 84; pattern of addiction, 6–7; pharmacological treatment, 85, 94–7; psychosocial treatment, 86–7; replacement therapy, 88–93
nicotine replacement therapy, 82, 85, 88: nicotine gum, 89; nicotine inhalers, 92; nicotine lozenges, 93; nicotine nasal spray, 91; nicotine patch, 90
nicotine vaccine, 85
nicotinic receptors, 14, 78–81
NMDA (N-methyl-d-aspartate) receptors, 26–7, 36, 37, 52, 129
norepinephrine (NE), 28, 30–3, 94, 101, 125
nucleus accumbens (NAc), reward system, 12–14, 16–22: action of opioids on, 62–3; actions of hallucinogens, 124–5; actions of marijuana on, 114; actions of nicotine on, 79; actions of stimulants on, 100; bupropion's effects, 94; implicated in relapse, 33

obesity, 154
obsessive compulsive disorder (OCD), 143, 146, 155

opioid receptors, 16, 37, 54, 63, 69, 70, 73, 147
opioids, 61: actions on reward circuits, 62; endogenous opioid neurotransmitters, 63; mechanism of dopamine increase, 14; pattern of addiction, 6–7; pharmacological treatment, 65, 68–73; psychosocial treatment for OUD, 66; screening for misuse of, 64; treatment settings, 67; withdrawal treatment, 74–5
orbitofrontal cortex (OFC), 19, 21, 25, 151

panic, 32, 116, 125
pharmacological treatment: for alcohol use disorder, 50, 52–7; for alcohol withdrawal syndrome (AWS), 58–9; for marijuana use disorder, 117; for opioid use disorder, 65; for stimulant use disorder, 107
phencyclidine (PCP), 128–9
precursor proteins, 63
prefrontal cortex (PFC), 13, 19, 21: and compulsive use/addiction, 24–5; and goal-directed behavior, 22; hypoactivity in impulsive aggression, 151; hypoactivity in obese patients, 154; and loss of control over drug use, 26–7
pregnancy: and nicotine replacement therapies, 88; and reduced-risk drinking, 49
prescription opioids, overdose from, 61
pro-opiomelanocortin (POMC), 63
pseudo-addiction, 2
psychiatric illness and comorbid substance use, treatment issues, 8–9
psychosocial treatment, 133–4: 12-step facilitation/fellowships, 141; for alcohol use disorder, 51; behavioral therapy, 136–7; cognitive behavioral therapy (CBT), 135–6; family therapy, 140; interpersonal therapy (IPT), 139; for marijuana use disorder, 118; motivational enhancement therapy (MET), 138; for nicotine dependence, 86–7; for opioid use disorder, 66; for stimulant use disorder, 108
pyromania, 148

reactive reward system, 18–19, 21, 27, 154
recommended drinking limits, 40
reduced-risk drinking, 48–9
reflective reward system, 19, 21–2, 25, 27
reinforcement, 4, 12, 16, 30: and alpha 4 beta 2 nicotine receptors, 80–1; and dopamine increase, 15, 103; and glutamatergic dysfunction, 27; mu receptors in the VTA, 63; substrates, 17
relapse, 33
reward circuits: activated in addiction, 28–9; dopamine mesolimbic pathway, 12–13; marijuana and THC actions on, 114; opioid actions on, 62; stimulant actions on, 100
risk factors: for addiction, 5; for relapse, 33

screening methods: alcohol use disorder, 42–3; opioid misuse, 64
sedative hypnotics, 122–3
serotonin (5HT), 16: and dysphoria, 32; and hallucinogens, 124–7; regulation of aggression, 151
SERT (serotonin transporter), 126–7
skin picking disorder, 155
smoking cessation: brief intervention, 83; management strategy, 84; nicotine replacement therapy, 88–93; pharmacological treatment, 85, 94–7; psychosocial treatment, 86–7
SSRIs (selective serotonin reuptake inhibitors), 50, 151–2
standard drinks, 38–9

stimulants, 99: abuse potential, 103; actions on reward circuits, 100; cocaethylene, 106; cocaine vs. methamphetamine, 101–2; effects and treatments, 105; experimental treatments, 110–11; mechanism of dopamine increase, 14; pattern of addiction, 6–7; pharmacological treatments, 107; progression of abuse, 104; psychosocial treatment, 108; synthetic, "bath salts," 131; withdrawal from, 109
stress: brain circuit implicated in addiction, 28, 29; during acute withdrawal, 31; neurotransmitters linked to, 32; relapse trigger, 27, 33; risk factor for addiction, 5, 33
striatum, 13, 15, 22–5
substance use disorders (SUDs): and comorbid psychiatric illness, 8–9; proposed DSM-V criteria, 3, 146; similarities with ICDs, 144–5
support groups, 141
synthetic drugs, 125, 131

telephone quit lines, smoking cessation, 87
temptation vs. willpower, 20–1
thalamus, 13, 22, 25
THC (delta-9-tetrahydrocannabinol), 114, 119
tolerance, 2, 6–7; development of, 30–1; hallucinogens, 127

topiramate, 50, 57, 59
trends for getting high, 130–1
trichotillomania (hair pulling disorder), 146, 155
tricyclic antidepressants (TCAs), 9, 50, 107
Twelve-Step Facilitation (TSF), 141
twelve-step fellowships, 141

vaccines: cocaine dependence, 110, 111; nicotine dependence, 85
varenicline, smoking cessation, 85, 96–7
ventral tegmental area (VTA), 12, 14, 16, 17, 28: actions of alcohol in, 36–7; actions of nicotine in, 78–9; and actions of opioids, 62–3; and drug-induced craving, 24–5; and loss of control over drug use, 27; reactive reward system, 18; and temptation, 20–1
ventromedial prefrontal cortex (VMPFC), 13, 19
vesicular monoamine transporter (VMAT), 102
voltage-sensitive calcium channels (VSCC), 36, 37

willpower vs. temptation, 20–1
withdrawal, 4: acute, mechanism of, 30–1; alcohol withdrawal syndrome, 58–9; marijuana, 119; motivational withdrawal syndrome, 32; opioids, symptoms of, 64; opioids, treatment of, 67, 74–5; stimulants, 109

Stahl's Illustrated

CME: Posttest and Certificate

Release/Expiration Dates
Release Date: October 1, 2012
CME Credit Expiration Date: September 30, 2015. *If this date has passed, please contact NEI for updated information.*

CME Posttest Study Guide

PLEASE NOTE: The posttest can only be submitted online. The posttest questions have been provided below solely as a study tool to prepare for your online submission. **Faxed/mailed copies of the posttest cannot be processed** and will be returned to the sender. If you do not have access to a computer, contact NEI customer service at 888-535-5600.

1. A 32-year-old man undergoing a standard screening for alcohol use states that he drinks 2-3 drinks a day, a couple of days a week. When asked to clarify, he says that a "drink" is typically a pint of beer. How many standard drinks is this patient consuming per week (assuming 2-3 "drinks" twice per week)?
   A. 4-6 drinks per week
   B. 5-8 drinks per week
   C. 8-12 drinks per week

2. A 73-year-old man presents to a new primary care provider for a routine physical exam. During the exam, he is asked some basic screening questions about alcohol use. The patient states that he drinks 1 mixed drink (containing a single 1-ounce shot) each night. How would you assess this patient's drinking behavior?
   A. Low-risk drinking
   B. At-risk drinking
   C. Alcohol use disorder

3. Mary is a 33-year-old woman with alcohol use disorder. She consumes several drinks a day nearly every day of the week and has recently had her two children removed from her care. She is motivated to attempt to stop drinking in order to get her children back. She previously attempted to quit cold turkey and on her own, and ended up in the emergency room with severe withdrawal symptoms. Considering these factors, would she be a good candidate for reduced-risk drinking as a goal?
   A. Yes
   B. No

Stahl's Illustrated

CME: Posttest and Certificate, continued

4. Todd is a 34-year-old man with a 10-year history of alcohol dependence, consuming 4-5 standard drinks a day, every day of the week. Due to some recent health problems, he decided to stop drinking and threw out all the alcohol in his home. Six hours later, he presents at urgent care with tremor, elevated pulse rate, sweating, agitation, and anxiety. Based on his presenting symptoms, does this patient need to be admitted?

   A. Yes, inpatient management is necessary
   B. No, outpatient management is appropriate for this patient

5. A 24-year-old woman with a 6-year history of smoking has decided that she is ready to quit. She is considering nicotine replacement therapy but is concerned that she may just end up dependent on that instead. Which of the available nicotine replacement therapies carries the highest risk of dependence?

   A. Gum
   B. Lozenge
   C. Nasal inhaler
   D. Nasal spray
   E. Transdermal patch

6. A 26-year-old woman develops a dependence on opioids after taking them during her recovery from knee surgery. She attempts to stop using them on her own, but when she does stop or decreases her dose she experiences nausea, muscle aches, sweating, diarrhea, insomnia, and depression. She and her practitioner decide that buprenorphine would be an appropriate treatment strategy. Which of the following is true?

   A. The patient should initiate buprenorphine while down-titrating her current opioid
   B. The patient should be in a mild withdrawal state prior to initiating buprenorphine
   C. The patient should complete withdrawal before beginning buprenorphine treatment

7. A 38-year-old man develops opioid dependence after taking an opioid during his recovery from back surgery. He is encouraged by his practitioner to attempt to stop the opioid. They decide that naltrexone along with appropriate nonpharmacological services is the best treatment for this patient with opioid dependence. Which of the following is true?

   A. The patient should initiate naltrexone before stopping his current opioid
   B. The patient should initiate naltrexone while down-titrating his current opioid
   C. The patient should be abstinent from his current opioid before beginning naltrexone treatment

8. A 23-year-old woman with opioid dependence is about to begin inpatient treatment to discontinue her opioid use. The treatment plan for this patient is to discontinue her opioid abruptly, using clonidine to suppress withdrawal symptoms. Which effects of clonidine can be expected?

   A. Reduction of vomiting, diarrhea, cramps, and sweating
   B. Reduction of insomnia, distress, and cravings
   C. Reduction of all these symptoms (vomiting, diarrhea, cramps, sweating, insomnia, distress, and cravings)

Stahl's Illustrated

CME: Posttest and Certificate, continued

9. A 26-year-old woman addicted to cocaine has reached the point at which she is ready to abstain. The accumulation of evidence supports the use of which of the following classes of agents to treat cocaine dependence?
   A. Anticonvulsants
   B. Antidepressants
   C. Dopamine agonists
   D. None of the above

10. A 26-year-old woman addicted to cocaine has reached the point at which she is ready to abstain. What can be expected in terms of withdrawal symptoms and associated treatment?
    A. Mild withdrawal requiring outpatient treatment
    B. Severe withdrawal requiring inpatient treatment

11. A 26-year-old woman with a history of marijuana use plans to become pregnant and has therefore decided to stop smoking marijuana. However, when she initially abstained, she developed emotional and behavioral symptoms suggestive of a withdrawal syndrome. What is the recommended pharmacotherapy for ameliorating the symptoms of marijuana withdrawal?
    A. Bupropion
    B. Divalproex
    C. Naltrexone
    D. There is no recommended pharmacotherapy for marijuana withdrawal

CME Online Posttest and Certificate
To receive your certificate of CME credit or participation, complete the posttest and activity evaluation available only online at **www.neiglobal.com/CME** (under "Book"). If a passing score of 70% or more is attained (required to receive credit), you can immediately print your certificate. There is a fee for the posttest (waived for NEI members). If you have questions or do not have access to a computer, contact customer service at 888-535-5600.